Virtual Clinical Excursions—Psychiatric

for

Stuart:
Principles and Practice of Psychiatric Nursing,
10th Edition

Virtual Clinical Excursions—Psychiatric

for

Stuart:
Principles and Practice of Psychiatric Nursing,
10th Edition

prepared by

Susan Fertig McDonald, DNP, PMHCNS-BC
Clinical Nurse Specialist—Psychiatry
VA San Diego Healthcare System
San Diego, California

software developed by

Wolfsong Informatics, LLC
Tucson, Arizona

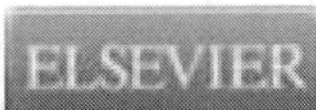

ELSEVIER
MOSBY

3251 Riverport Lane
Maryland Heights, Missouri 63043

VIRTUAL CLINICAL EXCURSIONS—PSYCHIATRIC FOR STUART: PRINCIPLES AND PRACTICE OF PSYCHIATRIC NURSING, TENTH EDITION

ISBN 978-0-323-10184-4

Notice

Knowledge and best practice in this field are constantly changing. As new research and experience broaden our understanding, changes in research methods, professional practices, or medical treatment may become necessary.

Practitioners and researchers must always rely on their own experience and knowledge in evaluating and using any information, methods, compounds, or experiments described herein. In using such information or methods they should be mindful of their own safety and the safety of others, including parties for whom they have a professional responsibility.

With respect to any drug or pharmaceutical products identified, readers are advised to check the most current information provided (i) on procedures featured or (ii) by the manufacturer of each product to be administered, to verify the recommended dose or formula, the method and duration of administration, and contraindications. It is the responsibility of practitioners, relying on their own experience and knowledge of their patients, to make diagnoses, to determine dosages and the best treatment for each individual patient, and to take all appropriate safety precautions.

To the fullest extent of the law, neither the Publisher nor the authors, contributors, or editors, assume any liability for any injury and/or damage to persons or property as a matter of products liability, negligence or otherwise, or from any use or operation of any methods, products, instructions, or ideas contained in the material herein.

ISBN 978-0-323-10184-4

Vice President, eSolutions – Nursing: *Tom Wilhelm*
Director, Simulation Solutions: *Jeff Downing*
Associate Content Development Specialist: *Sharifa Barakat*
Publishing Services Manager: *Jeff Patterson*
Senior Project Manager: *Tracey Schriefer*

Printed in the United States of America

Last digit is the print number: 9 8 7 6 5 4 3 2 1

Workbook
prepared by

Susan Fertig McDonald, DNP, PMHCNS-BC
Clinical Nurse Specialist—Psychiatry
VA San Diego Healthcare System
San Diego, California

Textbook

Gail Wiscarz Stuart, PhD, RN, FAAN
Dean and Distinguished University Professor, College of Nursing
Professor, College of Medicine
Department of Psychiatry and Behavioral Sciences
Medical University of South Carolina
Charleston, South Carolina

Contents

Table of Contents
Stuart:
Principles and Practice of Psychiatric Nursing, 10th Edition

Getting Started

GETTING SET UP

MINIMUM SYSTEM REQUIREMENTS

WINDOWS®

Windows Vista®, XP, 2000 (Recommend Windows XP/2000)
Pentium® III processor (or equivalent) @ 600 MHz (Recommend 800 MHz or better)
256 MB of RAM (Recommend 1 GB or more for Windows Vista)
800 x 600 screen size (Recommend 1024 x 768)
Thousands of colors
12x CD-ROM drive

Note: Windows Vista and XP require administrator privileges for installation.

MACINTOSH® (Note: This CD will not work in Mac Lion 10.7)

MAC OS X (up to 10.6)
Apple Power PC G3 @ 500 MHz or better
128 MB of RAM (Recommend 256 MB or more)
800 x 600 screen size (Recommend 1024 x 768)
Thousands of colors
12x CD-ROM drive
Stereo speakers or headphones

INSTALLATION INSTRUCTIONS

WINDOWS

1. Insert the *Virtual Clinical Excursions—Psychiatric* CD-ROM.
2. The setup screen should appear automatically if the current product is not already installed. Windows Vista users may be asked to authorize additional security prompts.
3. Follow the onscreen instructions during the setup process.

   If the setup screen does *not* appear automatically (and *Virtual Clinical Excursions—Psychiatric* has not been installed already):

   a. Click the **My Computer** icon on your desktop or on your Start menu.
   b. Double-click on your CD-ROM drive.
   c. If installation does not start at this point:
      (1) Click the **Start** icon on the taskbar and select the **Run** option.
      (2) Type d:\setup.exe (where "d:\" is your CD-ROM drive) and press **OK**.
      (3) Follow the onscreen instructions for installation.

MACINTOSH

1. Insert the *Virtual Clinical Excursions—Psychiatric* CD in the CD-ROM drive. The disk icon will appear on your desktop.
2. Double-click on the disk icon.
3. Double-click on the VCEPSYCH_MAC run file.

Note: Virtual Clinical Excursions—Psychiatric for Macintosh does not have an installation setup and can only be run directly from the CD.

HOW TO USE VIRTUAL CLINICAL EXCURSIONS—PSYCHIATRIC

WINDOWS

1. Double-click on the *Virtual Clinical Excursions—Psychiatric* icon located on your desktop.
2. Or navigate to the program via the Windows Start menu.

Note: If your computer uses Windows Vista, right-click on the desktop shortcut and choose **Properties**. In the Compatibility Mode, check the box for "Run as Administrator." Below is a screen capture to show what this looks like.

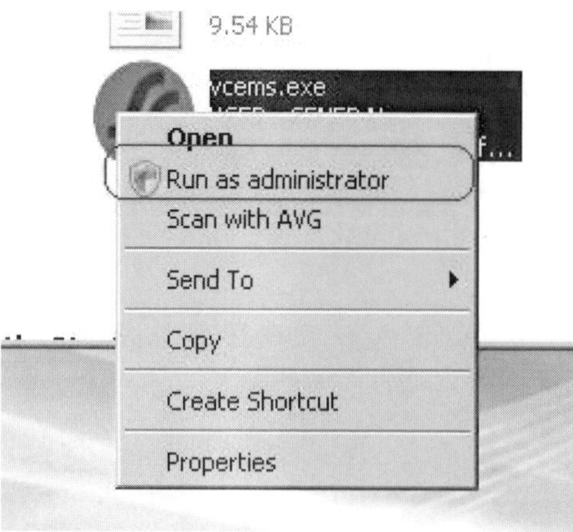

MACINTOSH

1. Insert the *Virtual Clinical Excursions—Psychiatric* CD in the CD-ROM drive. The disk icon will appear on your desktop.
2. Double-click on the disk icon.
3. Double-click on the VCEPSYCH_MAC run file.

SCREEN SETTINGS

For best results, your computer monitor resolution should be set at a minimum of 800 x 600. The number of colors displayed should be set to "thousands or higher" (High Color or 16 bit) or "millions of colors" (True Color or 24 bit).

Windows

1. From the **Start** menu, select **Control Panel** (on some systems, you will first go to **Settings**, then to **Control Panel**).
2. Double-click on the **Display** icon.
3. Click on the **Settings** tab.
4. Under **Screen resolution** use the slider bar to select **800 by 600 pixels**.
5. Access the **Colors** drop-down menu by clicking on the down arrow.
6. Select **High Color (16 bit)** or **True Color (24 bit)**.
7. Click on **OK**.
8. You may be asked to verify the setting changes. Click **Yes**.
9. You may be asked to restart your computer to accept the changes. Click **Yes**.

Macintosh

1. Select the **Monitors** control panel.
2. Select **800 x 600** (or similar) from the **Resolution** area.
3. Select **Thousands** or **Millions** from the **Color Depth** area.

WEB BROWSERS

Supported web browsers include Microsoft Internet Explorer (IE) version 7.0 or higher and Mozilla 3.0 or higher.

If you use America Online® (AOL) for web access, you will need AOL version 4.0 or higher and one of the browsers listed above. Do not use earlier versions of AOL with earlier versions of IE, because you will have difficulty accessing many features.

For best results with AOL:

- Connect to the Internet using AOL version 4.0 or higher.
- Open a private chat within AOL (this allows the AOL client to remain open, without asking whether you wish to disconnect while minimized).
- Minimize AOL.
- Launch a recommended browser.

TECHNICAL SUPPORT

Technical support for this product is available 24 hours a day, seven days a week, excluding holidays. Before calling, be sure that your computer meets the minimum system requirements to run this software. Inside the United States and Canada, call 1-800-222-9570. Outside North America, call 314-447-8094. You may also fax your questions to 314-447-8078 or contact Technical Support through e-mail: technical.support@elsevier.com.

Trademarks: Windows, Macintosh, Pentium, and America Online are registered trademarks.

ACCESSING *Virtual Clinical Excursions—Psychiatric* FROM EVOLVE

The product you have purchased is part of the Evolve family of online courses and learning resources. Please read the following information thoroughly to get started.

To access your instructor's course on Evolve:

Your instructor will provide you with the username and password needed to access this specific course on the Evolve Learning System. Once you have received this information, please follow these instructions:

1. Go to the Evolve student page (http://evolve.elsevier.com/student).
2. Enter your username and password in the **Login to My Evolve** area and click the **Login** button.
3. You will be taken to your personalized **My Evolve** page, where the course will be listed in the **My Courses** module.

TECHNICAL REQUIREMENTS

To use an Evolve course, you will need access to a computer that is connected to the Internet and equipped with web browser software that supports frames. For optimal performance, it is recommended that you have speakers and use a high-speed Internet connection. However, slower dial-up modems (56 K minimum) are acceptable.

Whichever browser you use, the browser preferences must be set to enable cookies and the cache must be set to reload every time.

Enable Cookies

Browser	Steps
Internet Explorer (IE) 7.0 or higher	1. Select **Tools → Internet Options**. 2. Select **Privacy** tab. 3. Use the slider (slide down) to **Accept All Cookies**. 4. Click **OK**. **-OR-** 3. Click the **Advanced** button. 4. Click the check box next to **Override Automatic Cookie Handling**. 5. Click the **Accept** radio buttons under **First-party Cookies** and **Third-party Cookies**. 6. Click **OK**.
Mozilla Firefox 3.0 or higher	1. Select **Tools → Options**. 2. Select the **Privacy** icon. 3. Click to expand Cookies. 4. Select **Allow sites to set cookies**. 5. Click **OK**.

Set Cache to Always Reload a Page

Browser	Steps
Internet Explorer (IE) 7.0 or higher	1. Select **Tools → Internet Options**. 2. Select **General** tab. 3. Go to the **Temporary Internet Files** and click the **Settings** button. 4. Select the radio button for **Every visit to the page** and click **OK** when complete.
Mozilla Firefox 3.0 or higher	1. Select **Tools → Options**. 2. Select the **Privacy** icon. 3. Click to expand Cache. 4. Set the value to "**0**" in the **Use up to: __ MB of disk space for the cache** field. 5. Click **OK**.

Plug-Ins

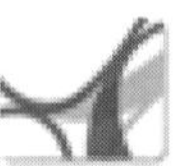

Adobe Acrobat Reader—With the free Acrobat Reader software, you can view and print Adobe PDF files. Many Evolve products offer student and instructor manuals, checklists, and more in this format!

Download at: http://www.adobe.com

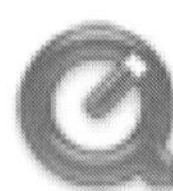

Apple QuickTime—Install this to hear word pronunciations, heart and lung sounds, and many other helpful audio clips within Evolve Online Courses!

Download at: http://www.apple.com

Adobe Flash Player—This player will enhance your viewing of many Evolve web pages, as well as educational short-form to long-form animation within the Evolve Learning System!

Download at: http://www.adobe.com

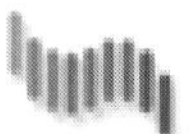

Adobe Shockwave Player—Shockwave is best for viewing the many interactive learning activities within Evolve Online Courses!

Download at: http://www.adobe.com

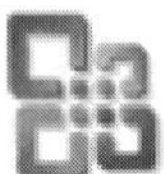

Microsoft Word Viewer—With this viewer, Microsoft Word users can share documents with those who don't have Word, and users without Word can open and view Word documents. Many Evolve products have testbank, student and instructor manuals, and other documents available for downloading and viewing on your own computer!

Download at: http://www.microsoft.com

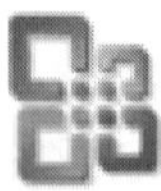

Microsoft PowerPoint Viewer—With this viewer, you can access PowerPoint 97, 2000, and 2002 presentations even if you don't have PowerPoint. Many Evolve products have slides available for downloading and viewing on your own computer!

Download at: http://www.microsoft.com

SUPPORT INFORMATION

Live phone support is available to customers in the United States and Canada at **800-222-9570** 24 hours a day, seven days a week, excluding holidays. Support is also available through email at technical.support@elsevier.com.

Online 24/7 support can be accessed on the Evolve website (http://evolve.elsevier.com). Resources include:

- Guided tours
- Tutorials
- Frequently asked questions (FAQs)
- Online copies of course user guides
- And much more!

A QUICK TOUR

Welcome to *Virtual Clinical Excursions—Psychiatric*, a virtual hospital setting in which you can work with multiple complex patient simulations and also learn to access and evaluate the information resources that are essential for high-quality patient care. The virtual hospital, Pacific View Regional Hospital, has realistic architecture and access to patient rooms, a Nurses' Station, and a Medication Room.

BEFORE YOU START

Make sure you have your textbook nearby when you use the *Virtual Clinical Excursions—Psychiatric* CD. You will want to consult topic areas in your textbook frequently while working with the CD and using this workbook.

HOW TO SIGN IN

- Enter your name on the Student Nurse identification badge.
- Next, click the down arrow next to **Select Floor**. This drop-down menu lists only the floors on which there are currently patients with psychiatric nursing needs: Medical-Surgical, Obstetrics, Pediatrics, and Skilled Nursing. (For this quick tour, choose **Obstetrics**.)
- Now choose one of the four periods of care in which to work. In Periods of Care 1 through 3, you can actively engage in patient assessment, entry of data in the electronic patient record (EPR), and medication administration. Period of Care 4 presents the day in review. Highlight and click the appropriate period of care. (For this quick tour, choose **Period of Care 1**.)
- Click **Go**. This takes you to the Patient List screen (see example on page 11). Note that the virtual time is provided in the box at the lower left corner of the screen (0730, since we chose Period of Care 1).

Note: If you choose to work during Period of Care 4: 1900-2000, the Patient List screen is skipped since you are not able to visit patients or administer medications during the shift. Instead, you are taken directly to the Nurses' Station, where the records of all the patients on the floor are available for your review.

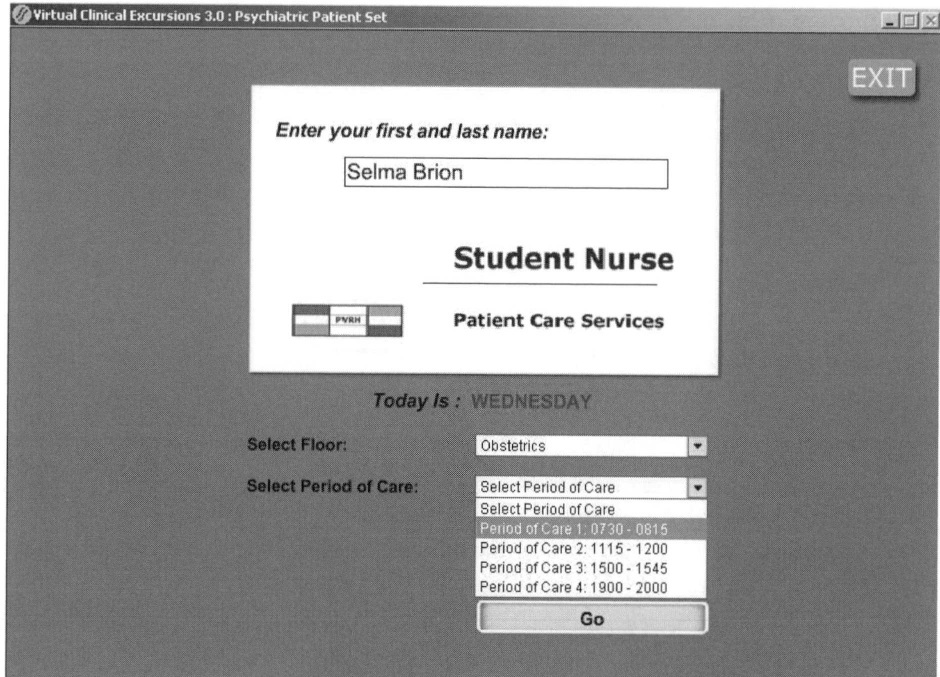

PATIENT LIST

OBSTETRICS UNIT

Dorothy Grant (Room 201)
30-week intrauterine pregnancy—A 25-year-old Caucasian multipara admitted with abdominal trauma following a domestic violence incident. Her complications include preterm labor and extensive social issues such as acquiring safe housing for her family upon discharge.

Kelly Brady (Room 203)
26-week intrauterine pregnancy—A 35-year-old Caucasian primigravida urgently admitted for progressive symptoms of preeclampsia. A history of inadequate coping with major life stressors leave her at risk for a recurrence of depression as she faces a diagnosis of HELLP syndrome and the delivery of a severely premature infant.

Laura Wilson (Room 206)
37-week intrauterine pregnancy—An 18-year-old Caucasian primigravida urgently admitted after being found unconscious. Her complications include HIV-positive status and chronic polysubstance abuse. Unrealistic expectations of parenthood and living with a chronic illness, combined with strained family relations, prompt comprehensive social and psychiatric evaluations initiated on the day of simulation.

PEDIATRIC UNIT

Tiffany Sheldon (Room 305)
Anorexia nervosa—A 14-year-old Caucasian female admitted for dehydration, electrolyte imbalance, and malnutrition following a syncope episode at home. This patient has a history of eating disorders that have required multiple hospital admissions and have strained family dynamics between mother and daughter.

MEDICAL-SURGICAL UNIT

Harry George (Room 401)
Osteomyelitis—A 54-year-old Caucasian male admitted from a homeless shelter with an infected leg. He has complications of type 2 diabetes mellitus, alcohol abuse, nicotine addiction, poor pain control, and complex psychosocial issues.

Jacquline Catanazaro (Room 402)
Asthma—A 45-year-old Caucasian female admitted with an acute asthma exacerbation and suspected pneumonia. She has complications of chronic schizophrenia, noncompliance with medication therapy, obesity, and herniated disk.

SKILLED NURSING UNIT

Kathryn Doyle (Room 503)
Rehabilitation post left hip replacement—A 79-year-old Caucasian female admitted following a complicated recovery from an ORIF. She is experiencing symptoms of malnutrition and depression due to unstable family dynamics, placing her at risk for elder abuse.

Carlos Reyes (Room 504)
Rehabilitation status post myocardial infarction—An 81-year-old Hispanic male admitted for evaluation of the need for long-term care following an acute care hospital stay. Recent cognitive changes and a diagnosis of anxiety disorder contribute to stressful family dynamics and caregiver strain.

HOW TO SELECT A PATIENT

- You can choose one or more patients to work with from the Patient List by checking the box to the left of the patient name(s). For this quick tour, select Dorothy Grant. (In order to receive a scorecard for a patient, the patient must be selected before proceeding to the Nurses' Station.)
- Click on **Get Report** to the right of the medical records number (MRN) to view a summary of the patient's care during the 12-hour period before your arrival on the unit.
- After reviewing the report, click on **Go to Nurses' Station** in the right lower corner to begin your care. (*Note:* If you have been assigned to care for multiple patients, you can click on **Return to Patient List** to select and review the report for each additional patient before going to the Nurses' Station.)

Note: Even though the Patient List is initially skipped when you sign in to work for Period of Care 4, you can still access this screen if you wish to review the shift report for any of the patients. To do so, simply click on **Patient List** near the top left corner of the Nurses' Station (or click on the clipboard to the left of the Kardex). Then click on **Get Report** for the patient(s) whose care you are reviewing. This may be done during any period of care.

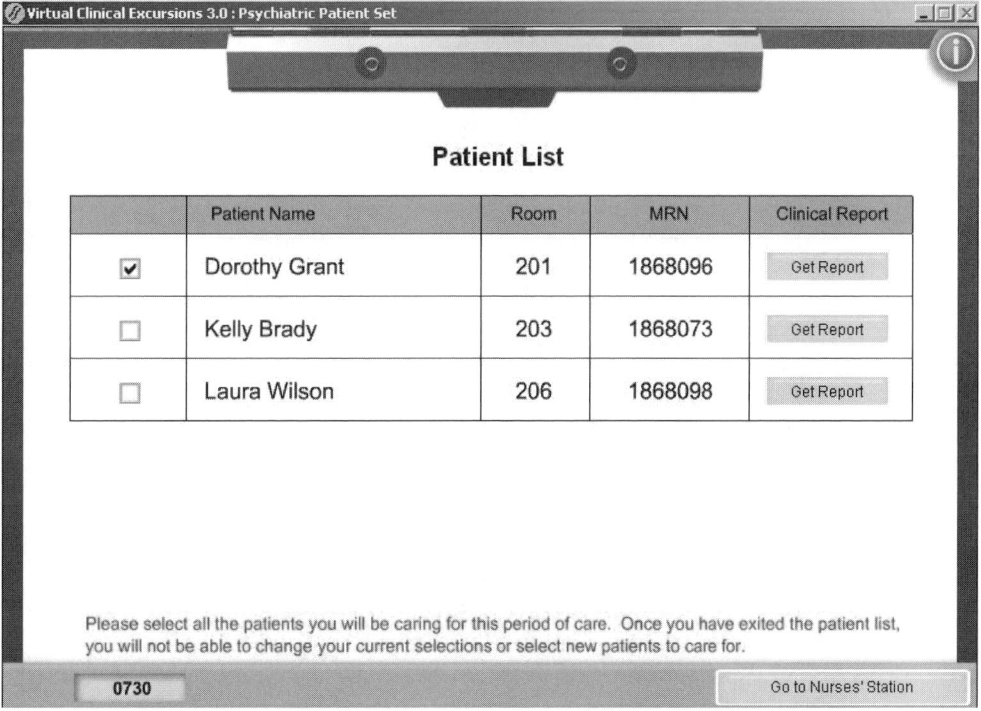

HOW TO FIND A PATIENT'S RECORDS

NURSES' STATION

Within the Nurses' Station, you will see:

1. A clipboard that contains the patient list for that floor.
2. A chart rack with patient charts labeled by room number, a notebook labeled Kardex, and a notebook labeled MAR (Medication Administration Record).
3. A desktop computer with access to the Electronic Patient Record (EPR).
4. A tool bar across the top of the screen that can also be used to access the Patient List, EPR, Chart, MAR, and Kardex. This tool bar is also accessible from each patient's room.
5. A Drug Guide containing information about the medications you are able to administer to your patients.
6. A tool bar across the bottom of the screen that can be used to access the Floor Map, patient rooms, Medication Room, and Drug Guide.

As you run your cursor over an item, it will be highlighted. To select, simply double-click on the item. As you use these resources, you will always be able to return to the Nurses' Station by clicking on the **Return to Nurses' Station** bar located in the right lower corner of your screen.

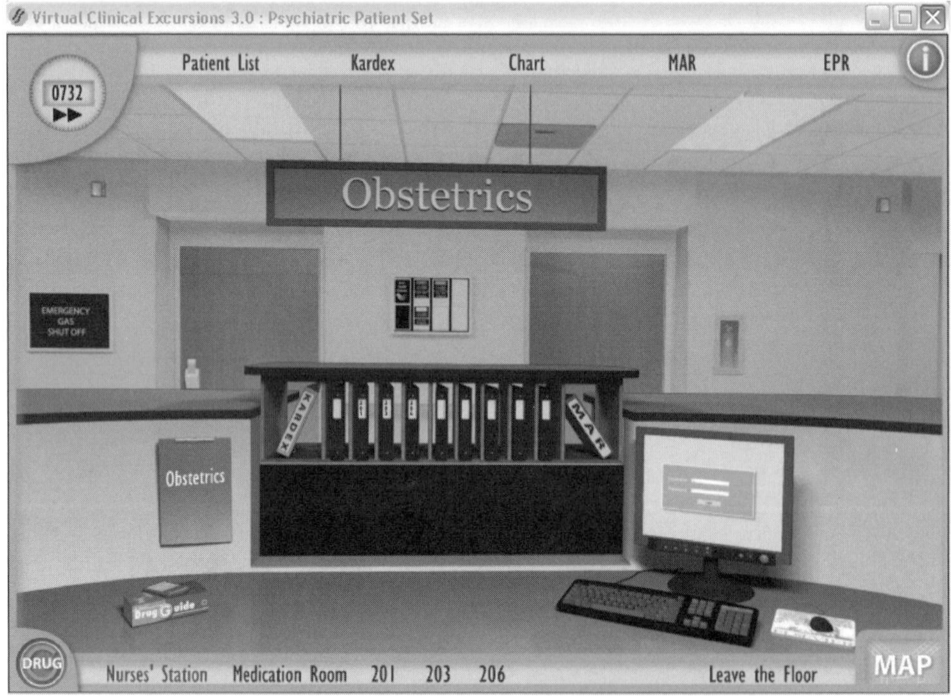

MEDICATION ADMINISTRATION RECORD (MAR)

The MAR icon located on the tool bar at the top of your screen accesses current 24-hour medications for each patient. Click on the icon and the MAR will open. (*Note:* You can also access the MAR by clicking on the MAR notebook on the far right side of the book rack in the center of the screen.) Within the MAR, tabs on the right side of the screen allow you to select patients by room number. Be careful to make sure you select the correct tab number for *your* patient rather than simply reading the first record that appears after the MAR opens. Each MAR sheet lists the following:

- Medications
- Route and dosage of each medication
- Times of administration of each medication

Note: The MAR changes each day. Expired MARs are stored in the patients' charts.

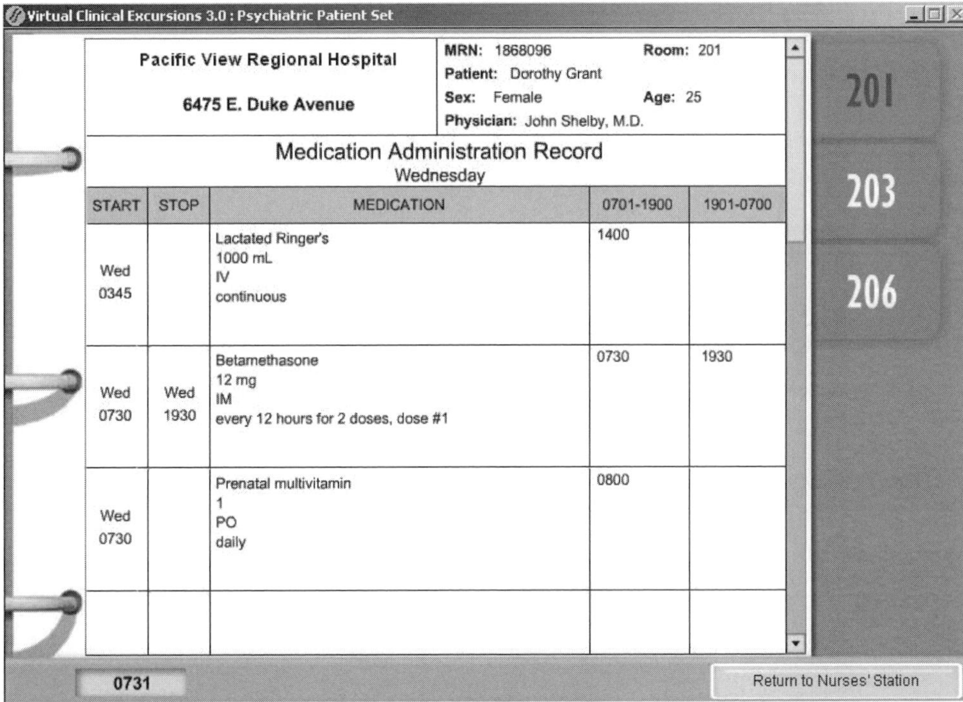

CHARTS

To access patient charts, either click on the **Chart** icon at the top of your screen or anywhere within the chart rack in the center of the Nurses' Station screen. When the close-up view appears, the individual charts are labeled by room number. To open a chart, click on the room number of the patient whose chart you wish to review. The patient's name and allergies will appear on the left side of the screen, along with a list of tabs on the right side of the screen, allowing you to view the following data:

- Allergies
- Physician's Orders
- Physician's Notes
- Nurse's Notes
- Laboratory Reports
- Diagnostic Reports
- Surgical Reports
- Consultations
- Patient Education
- History and Physical
- Nursing Admission
- Expired MARs
- Consents
- Mental Health
- Admissions
- Emergency Department

Information appears in real time. The entries are in reverse chronologic order, so use the down arrow at the right side of each chart page to scroll down to view previous entries. Flip from tab to tab to view multiple data fields or click on **Return to Nurses' Station** in the lower right corner of the screen to exit the chart.

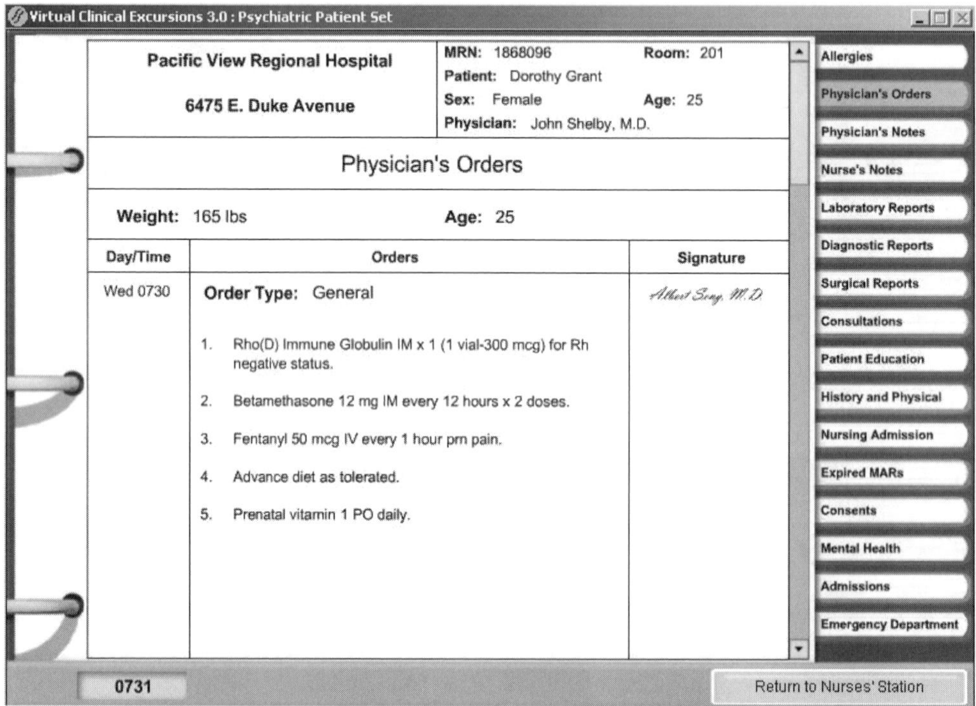

ELECTRONIC PATIENT RECORD (EPR)

The EPR can be accessed from the computer in the Nurses' Station or from the EPR icon located in the tool bar at the top of your screen. To access a patient's EPR:

- Click on either the computer screen or the **EPR** icon.
- Your username and password are automatically filled in.
- Click on **Login** to enter the EPR.
- *Note:* Like the MAR, the EPR is arranged numerically. Thus when you enter, you are initially shown the records of the patient in the lowest room number on the floor. To view the correct data for *your* patient, remember to select the correct room number, using the drop-down menu for the Patient field at the top left corner of the screen.

The EPR used in Pacific View Regional Hospital represents a composite of commercial versions being used in hospitals. You can access the EPR:

- to review existing data for a patient (by room number).
- to enter data you collect while working with a patient.

The EPR is updated daily, so no matter what day or part of a shift you are working, there will be a current EPR with the patient's data from the past days of the current hospital stay. This type of simulated EPR allows you to examine how data for different attributes have changed over time, as well as to examine data for all of a patient's attributes at a particular time. The EPR is fully functional (as it is in a real-life hospital). You can enter such data as blood pressure, breath sounds, and certain treatments. The EPR will not, however, allow you to enter data for a previous time period. Use the arrows at the bottom of the screen to move forward and backward in time.

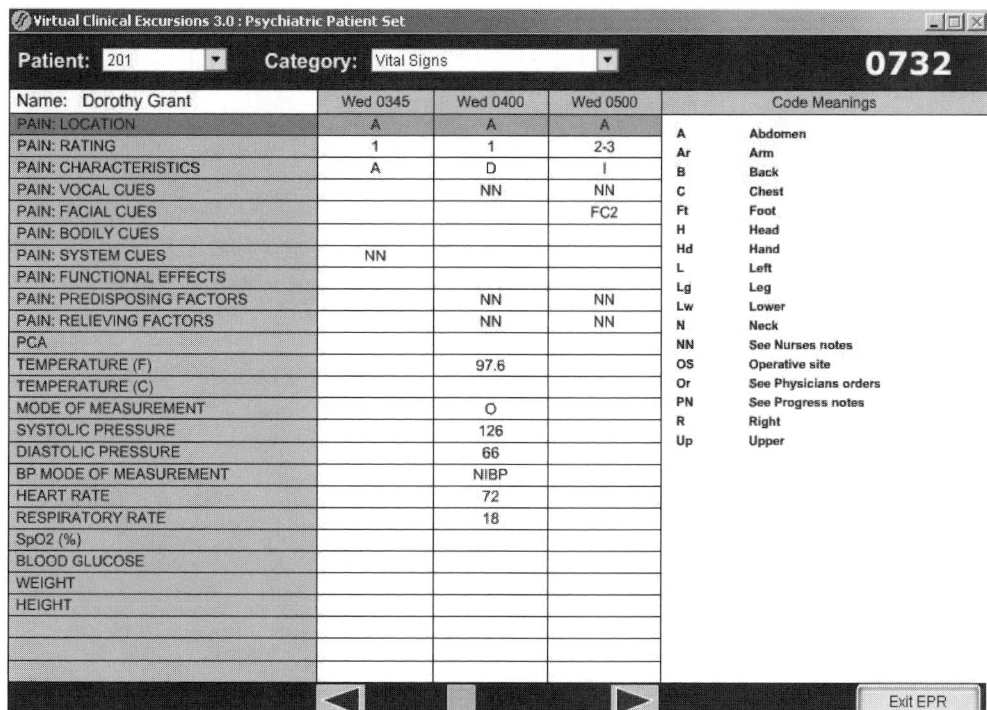

Virtual Clinical Excursions 3.0 : Psychiatric Patient Set

Patient: 201 Category: Vital Signs 0732

Name: Dorothy Grant	Wed 0345	Wed 0400	Wed 0500
PAIN: LOCATION	A	A	A
PAIN: RATING	1	1	2-3
PAIN: CHARACTERISTICS	A	D	I
PAIN: VOCAL CUES		NN	NN
PAIN: FACIAL CUES			FC2
PAIN: BODILY CUES			
PAIN: SYSTEM CUES	NN		
PAIN: FUNCTIONAL EFFECTS			
PAIN: PREDISPOSING FACTORS		NN	NN
PAIN: RELIEVING FACTORS		NN	NN
PCA			
TEMPERATURE (F)		97.6	
TEMPERATURE (C)			
MODE OF MEASUREMENT		O	
SYSTOLIC PRESSURE		126	
DIASTOLIC PRESSURE		66	
BP MODE OF MEASUREMENT		NIBP	
HEART RATE		72	
RESPIRATORY RATE		18	
SpO2 (%)			
BLOOD GLUCOSE			
WEIGHT			
HEIGHT			

Code Meanings	
A	Abdomen
Ar	Arm
B	Back
C	Chest
Ft	Foot
H	Head
Hd	Hand
L	Left
Lg	Leg
Lw	Lower
N	Neck
NN	See Nurses notes
OS	Operative site
Or	See Physicians orders
PN	See Progress notes
R	Right
Up	Upper

Exit EPR

At the top of the EPR screen, you can choose patients by their room numbers. In addition, you have access to 17 different categories of patient data. To change patients or data categories, click the down arrow to the right of the room number or category.

The categories of patient data in the EPR are as follows:

- Vital Signs
- Respiratory
- Cardiovascular
- Neurologic
- Gastrointestinal
- Excretory
- Musculoskeletal
- Integumentary
- Reproductive
- Psychosocial
- Wounds and Drains
- Activity
- Hygiene and Comfort
- Safety
- Nutrition
- IV
- Intake and Output

Remember, each hospital selects its own codes. The codes used in the EPR at Pacific View Regional Hospital may be different from ones you have seen in your clinical rotations. Take some time to acquaint yourself with the codes. Within the Vital Signs category, click on any item in the left column (e.g., Pain: Characteristics). In the far-right column, you will see a list of code meanings for the possible findings and/or descriptors for that assessment area.

You will use the codes to record the data you collect as you work with patients. Click on the box in the last time column to the right of any item and wait for the code meanings applicable to that entry to appear. Select the appropriate code to describe your assessment findings and type it in the box. (*Note:* If no cursor appears within the box, click on the box again until the blue shading disappears and the blinking cursor appears.) Once the data are typed in this box, they are entered into the patient's record for this period of care only.

To leave the EPR, click on **Exit EPR** in the bottom right corner of the screen.

VISITING A PATIENT

From the Nurses' Station, click on the room number of the patient you wish to visit (in the tool bar at the bottom of your screen). Once you are inside the room, you will see a still photo of your patient in the top left corner. To verify that this is the correct patient, click on the **Check Armband** icon to the right of the photo. The patient's identification data will appear. If you click on **Check Allergies** (the next icon to the right), a list of the patient's allergies (if any) will replace the photo.

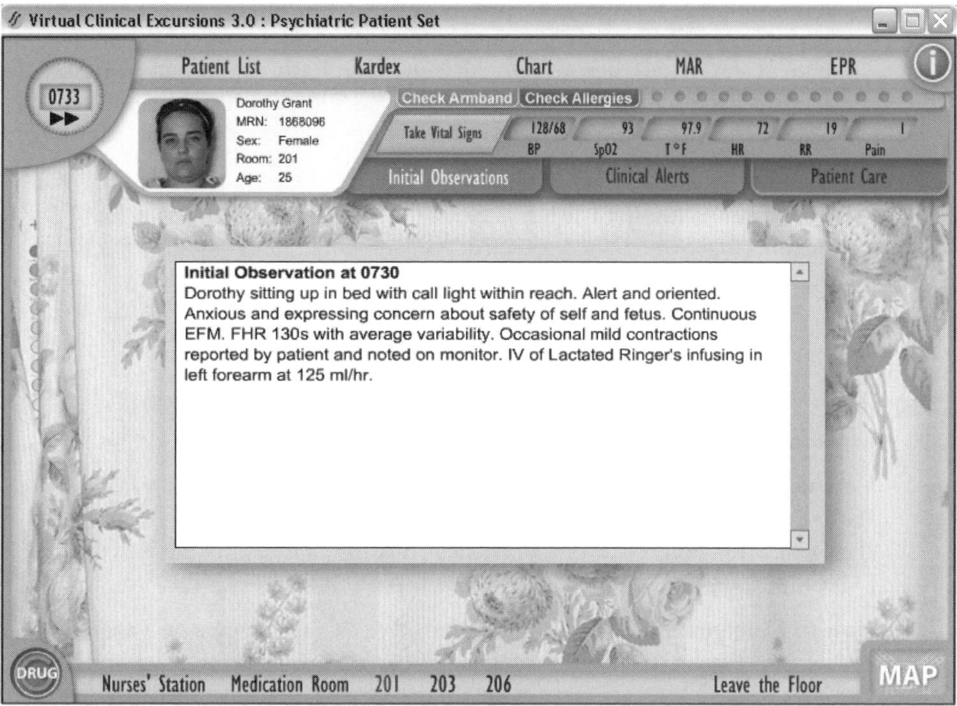

Also located in the patient's room are multiple icons you can use to assess the patient or the patient's medications. A virtual clock is provided in the upper left corner of the room to monitor your progress in real time. (*Note:* The fast-forward icon within the virtual clock will advance the time by 2-minute intervals when clicked.)

- The tool bar across the top of the screen allows you to check the **Patient List**, access the **EPR** to check or enter data, and view the patient's **Chart**, **MAR**, or **Kardex**.
- The **Take Vital Signs** icon allows you to measure the patient's up-to-the-minute blood pressure, oxygen saturation, temperature, heart rate, respiratory rate, and pain level.
- Each time you enter a patient's room, you are given an Initial Observation report to review (in the text box under the patient's photo). These notes are provided to give you a "look" at the patient as if you had just stepped into the room. You can also click on the **Initial Observations** icon to return to this box from other views within the patient's room. To the right of this icon is **Clinical Alerts**, a resource that allows you to make decisions about priority medication interventions based on emerging data collected in real time. Check this screen throughout your period of care to avoid missing critical information related to recently ordered or STAT medications.
- Clicking on **Patient Care** opens up three specific learning environments within the patient room: **Physical Assessment**, **Nurse-Client Interactions**, and **Medication Administration**.
- To perform a **Physical Assessment**, choose a body area (such as **Head & Neck**) from the column of yellow buttons. This activates a list of system subcategories for that body area (e.g., see **Sensory**, **Neurologic**, etc. in the green boxes). After you select the system you

wish to evaluate, a brief description of the assessment findings will appear in a box to the right. A still photo provides a "snapshot" of how an assessment of this area might be done or what the finding might look like. For every body area, you can also click on **Equipment** on the right side of the screen.

- To the right of the Physical Assessment icon is **Nurse-Client Interactions**. Clicking on this icon will reveal the times and titles of any videos available for viewing. (*Note:* If the video you wish to see is not listed, this means you have not yet reached the correct virtual time to view that video. Check the virtual clock; you may return to access the video once its designated time has occurred—as long as you do so within the same period of care. Or you can click on the fast-forward icon within the virtual clock to advance the time by 2-minute intervals. You will then need to click again on **Patient Care** and **Nurse-Client Interactions** to refresh the screen.) To view a listed video, click on the white arrow to the right of the video title. Use the control buttons below the video to start, stop, pause, rewind, or fast-forward the action or to mute the sound.

- **Medication Administration** is the pathway that allows you to review and administer medications to a patient after you have prepared them in the Medication Room. This process is addressed further in the *How to Prepare Medications* section (pages 19-20) and in *Medications* (pages 26-30). For additional hands-on practice, see *Reducing Medication Errors* (pages 37-41).

HOW TO QUIT, CHANGE PATIENTS, CHANGE FLOORS, OR CHANGE PERIODS OF CARE

How to Quit: From most screens, you may click the **Leave the Floor** icon on the bottom tool bar to the right of the patient room numbers. (*Note:* From some screens, you will first need to click an **Exit** button or **Return to Nurses' Station** before clicking **Leave the Floor**.) When the Floor Menu appears, click **Exit** to leave the program.

How to Change Patients, Floors, or Periods of Care: To change patients, simply click on the new patient's room number. (You cannot receive a scorecard for a new patient, however, unless you have already selected that patient on the Patient List screen.) To change to a new period of care, to change floors, or to restart the virtual clock, click on **Leave the Floor** and then on **Restart the Program**.

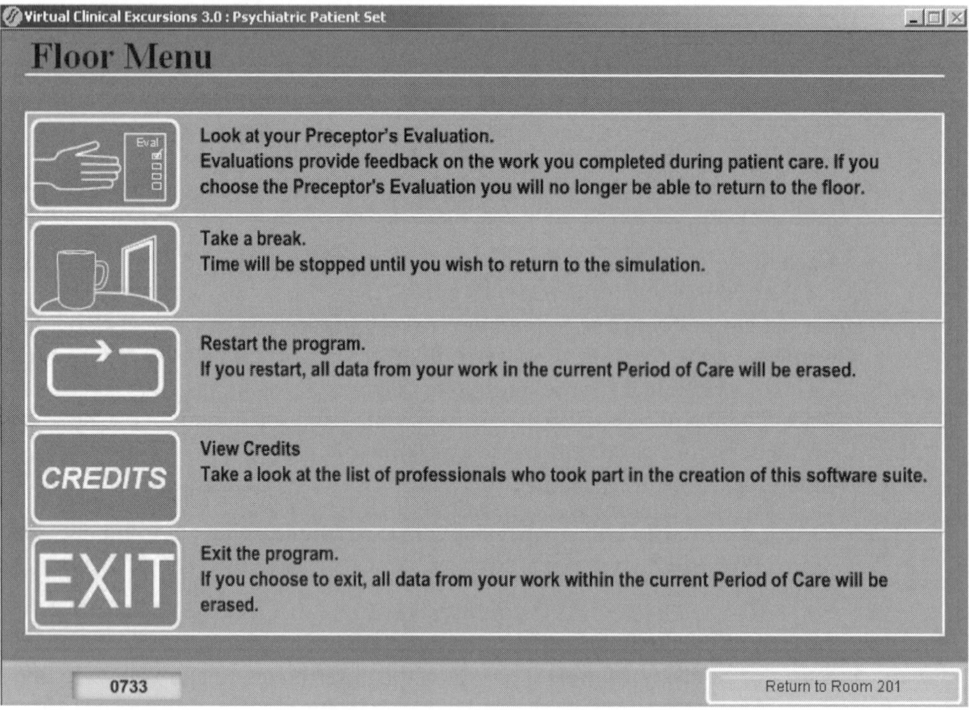

HOW TO PREPARE MEDICATIONS

From the Nurses' Station or the patient's room, you can access the Medication Room by clicking on the icon in the tool bar at the bottom of your screen to the left of the patient room numbers.

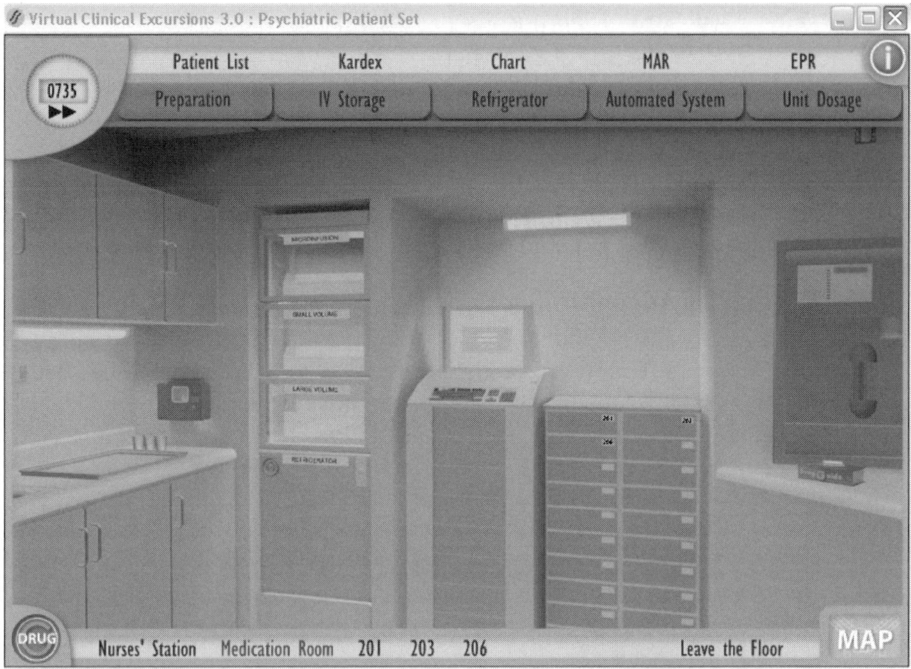

In the Medication Room you have access to the following (from left to right):

- A preparation area is located on the counter under the cabinets. To begin the medication preparation process, click on the tray on the counter or click on the **Preparation** icon at the top of the screen. The next screen leads you through a specific sequence (called the Preparation Wizard) to prepare medications one at a time for administration to a patient. However, no medication has been selected at this time. We will do this while working with a patient in *A Detailed Tour*. To exit this screen, click on **View Medication Room**.

- To the right of the cabinets (and above the refrigerator), IV storage bins are provided. Click on the bins themselves or on the **IV Storage** icon at the top of the screen. The bins are labeled **Microinfusion**, **Small Volume**, and **Large Volume**. Click on an individual bin to see a list of its contents. If you needed to prepare an IV medication at this time, you could click on the medication and its label would appear to the right under the patient's name. (*Note:* You can **Open** and **Close** any medication label by clicking the appropriate icon.) Next, you would click **Put Medication on Tray**. If you ever change your mind or decide that you have put the incorrect medication on the tray, you can reverse your actions by highlighting the medication on the tray and then clicking **Put Medication in Bin**. Click **Close Bin** in the right bottom corner to exit. **View Medication Room** brings you back to a full view of the entire room.

- A refrigerator is located under the IV storage bins to hold any medications that must be stored below room temperature. Click on the refrigerator door or on the **Refrigerator** icon at the top of the screen. Then click on the close-up view of the door to access the medications. When you are finished, click **Close Door** and then **View Medication Room**.

- To prepare controlled substances, click the **Automated System** icon at the top of the screen or click the computer monitor located to the right of the IV storage bins. A login screen will appear; your name and password are automatically filled in. Click **Login**. Select the patient for whom you wish to access medications; then select the correct medication drawer to open (they are stored alphabetically). Click **Open Drawer**, highlight the proper medication, and choose **Put Medication on Tray**. When you are finished, click **Close Drawer** and then **View Medication Room**.

- Next to the Automated System is a set of drawers identified by patient room number. To access these, click on the drawers or on the **Unit Dosage** icon at the top of the screen. This provides a close-up view of the drawers. To open a drawer, click on the room number of the patient you are working with. Next, click on the medication you would like to prepare for the patient, and a label will appear, listing the medication strength, units, and dosage per unit. To exit, click **Close Drawer**; then click **View Medication Room**.

At any time, you can learn about a medication you wish to prepare for a patient by clicking on the **Drug** icon in the bottom left corner of the medication room screen or by clicking the **Drug Guide** book on the counter to the right of the unit dosage drawers. The **Drug Guide** provides information about the medications commonly included in nursing drug handbooks. Nutritional supplements and maintenance intravenous fluid preparations are not included. Highlight a medication in the alphabetical list; relevant information about the drug will appear in the screen below. To exit, click **Return to Medication Room**.

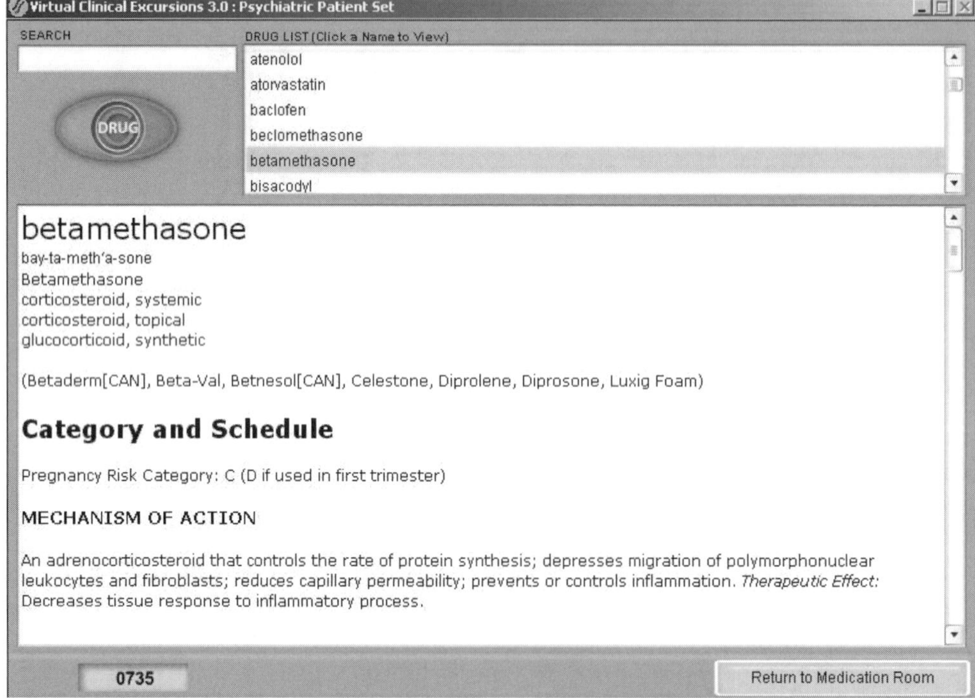

To access the MAR from the Medication Room and to review the medications ordered for a patient, click on the **MAR** icon located in the tool bar at the top of your screen and then click on the correct tab for your patient's room number. You may also click the **Review MAR** icon in the tool bar at the bottom of your screen from inside each medication storage area.

After you have chosen and prepared medications, go to the patient's room to administer them by clicking on the room number in the bottom tool bar. Inside the patient's room, click **Patient Care** and then **Medication Administration** and follow the proper administration sequence.

PRECEPTOR'S EVALUATIONS

When you have finished a session, click on **Leave the Floor** to go to the Floor Menu. At this point, you can click on the top icon (**Look at Your Preceptor's Evaluation**) to receive a scorecard that provides feedback on the work you completed during patient care.

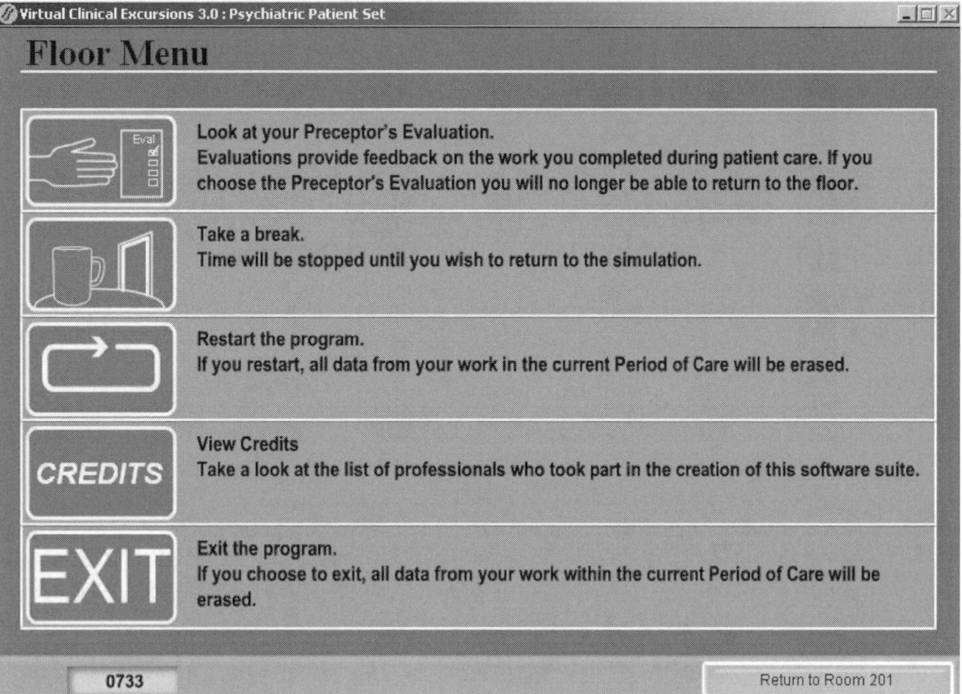

Evaluations are available for each patient you selected when you signed in for the current period of care. Click on the **Medication Scorecard** icon to see an example.

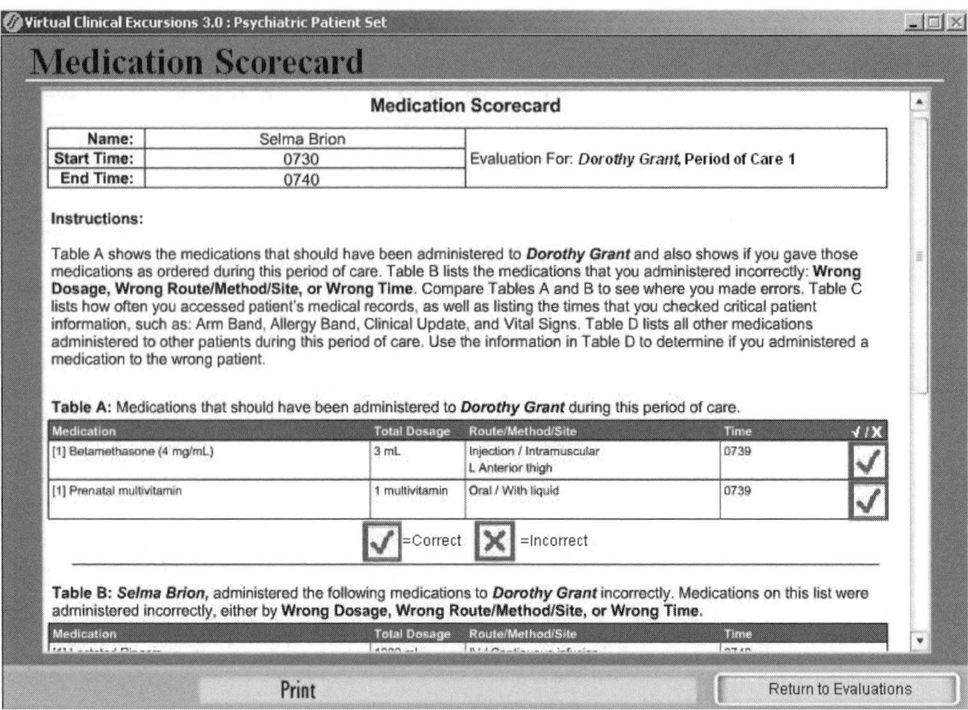
Virtual Clinical Excursions 3.0 : Psychiatric Patient Set

Medication Scorecard

Medication Scorecard

Name:	Selma Brion	Evaluation For: *Dorothy Grant*, **Period of Care 1**
Start Time:	0730	
End Time:	0740	

Instructions:

Table A shows the medications that should have been administered to ***Dorothy Grant*** and also shows if you gave those medications as ordered during this period of care. Table B lists the medications that you administered incorrectly: **Wrong Dosage, Wrong Route/Method/Site, or Wrong Time**. Compare Tables A and B to see where you made errors. Table C lists how often you accessed patient's medical records, as well as listing the times that you checked critical patient information, such as: Arm Band, Allergy Band, Clinical Update, and Vital Signs. Table D lists all other medications administered to other patients during this period of care. Use the information in Table D to determine if you administered a medication to the wrong patient.

Table A: Medications that should have been administered to ***Dorothy Grant*** during this period of care.

Medication	Total Dosage	Route/Method/Site	Time	√/X
[1] Betamethasone (4 mg/mL)	3 mL	Injection / Intramuscular L Anterior thigh	0739	√
[1] Prenatal multivitamin	1 multivitamin	Oral / With liquid	0739	√

√ =Correct X =Incorrect

Table B: ***Selma Brion,*** administered the following medications to ***Dorothy Grant*** incorrectly. Medications on this list were administered incorrectly, either by **Wrong Dosage, Wrong Route/Method/Site, or Wrong Time.**

Medication	Total Dosage	Route/Method/Site	Time

Print

Return to Evaluations

The scorecard compares the medications you administered to a patient during a period of care with what should have been administered. Table A lists the correct medications. Table B lists any medications that were administered incorrectly.

Remember, not every medication listed on the MAR should necessarily be given. For example, a patient might have an allergy to a drug that was ordered, or a medication might have been improperly transcribed to the MAR. Predetermined medication "errors" embedded within the program challenge you to exercise critical thinking skills and professional judgment when deciding to administer a medication, just as you would in a real hospital. Use all your available resources, such as the patient's chart and the MAR, to make your decision.

Table C lists the resources that were available to assist you in medication administration. It also documents whether and when you accessed these resources. For example, did you check the patient armband or perform a check of vital signs? If so, when?

You can click **Print** to get a copy of this report if needed. When you have finished reviewing the scorecard, click **Return to Evaluations** and then **Return to Menu**.

FLOOR MAP

To get a general sense of your location within the hospital, you can click on the **Map** icon found in the lower right corner of most of the screens in the *Virtual Clinical Excursions—Psychiatric* program. (*Note:* If you are following this quick tour step by step, you will need to **Restart the Program** from the Floor Menu, sign in again, and go to the Nurses' Station to access the map.) When you click the **Map** icon, a floor map appears, showing the layout of the floor you are currently on, as well as a directory of the patients and services on that floor. As you move your cursor over the directory list, the location of each room is highlighted on the map (and vice versa). The floor map can be accessed from the Nurses' Station, Medication Room, and each patient's room.

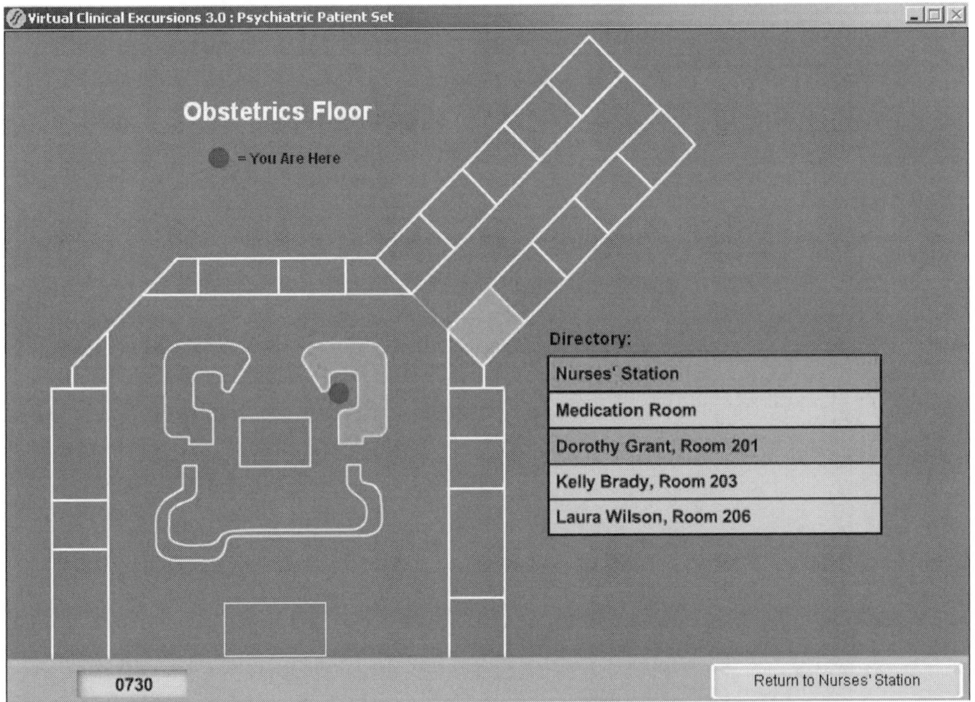

A DETAILED TOUR

If you wish to more thoroughly understand the capabilities of *Virtual Clinical Excursions—Psychiatric*, take a detailed tour by completing the following section. During this tour, we will work with a specific patient to introduce you to all the different components and learning opportunities available within the software.

WORKING WITH A PATIENT

Sign in and select the Obstetrics Floor for Period of Care 1 (0730-0815). From the Patient List, select Dorothy Grant in Room 201; however, do not go to the Nurses' Station yet.

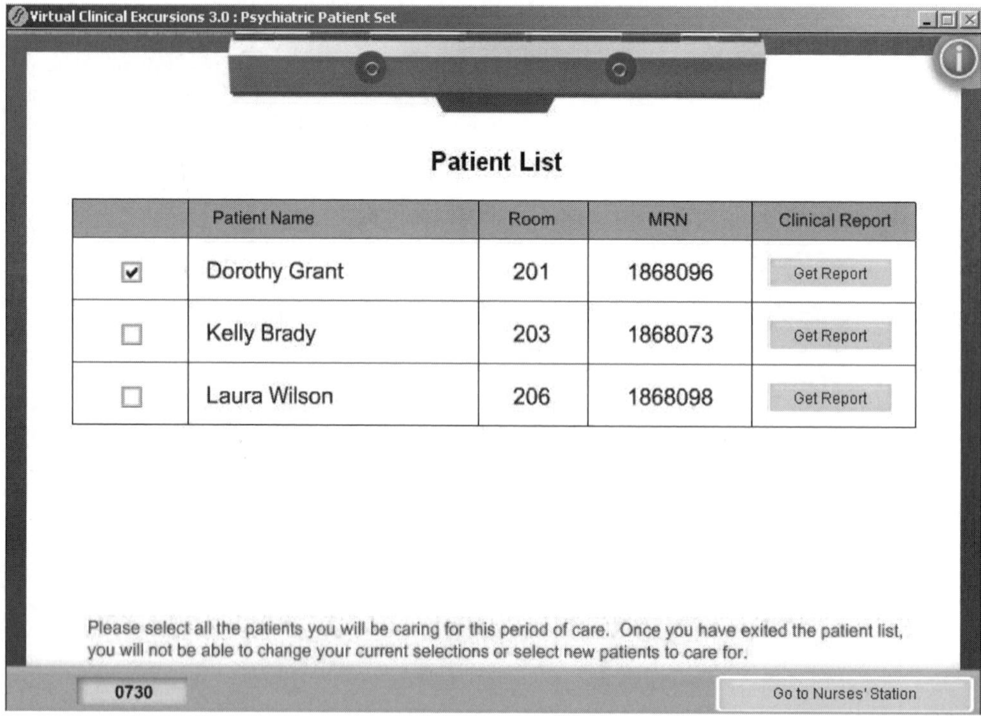

REPORT

In hospitals, when one shift ends and another begins, the outgoing nurse who attended a patient will give a verbal and sometimes a written summary of that patient's condition to the incoming nurse who will assume care for the patient. This summary is called a report and is an important source of data to provide an overview of a patient. Your first task is to get the clinical report on Dorothy Grant. To do this, click **Get Report** in the far right column in this patient's row. From a brief review of this summary, identify the problems and areas of concern that you will need to address for this patient.

When you have finished noting any areas of concern, click on **Go to Nurses' Station**.

CHARTS

You can access Dorothy Grant's chart from the Nurses' Station or from the patient's room (201). From the Nurses' Station, click on the chart rack or on the **Chart** icon in the tool bar at the top of your screen. Next, click on the chart labeled **201** to open the medical record for Dorothy Grant. Click on the **Emergency Department** tab to view a record of why this patient was admitted.

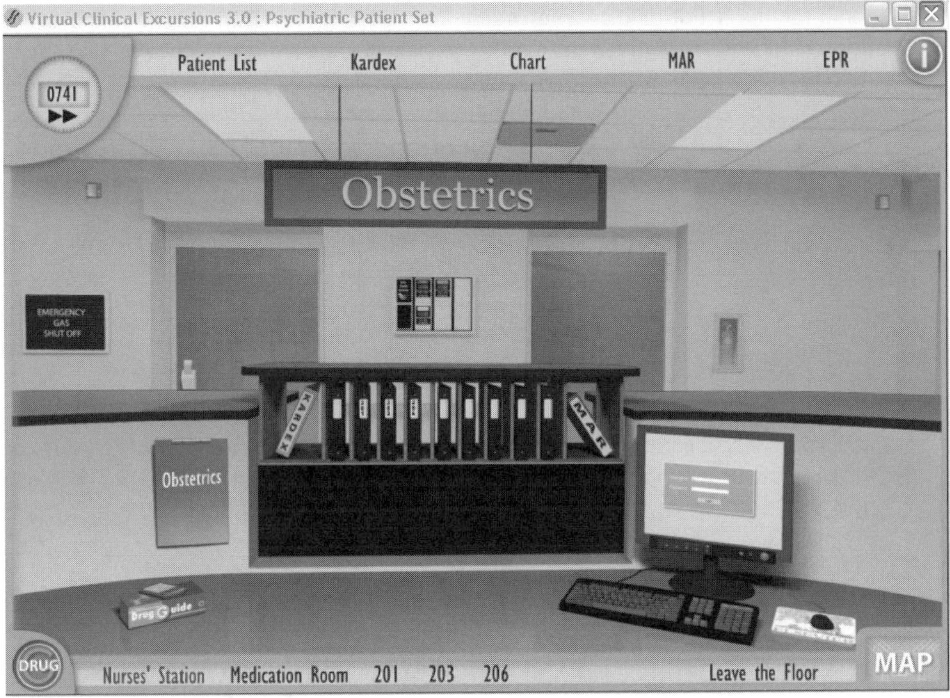

How many days has Dorothy Grant been in the hospital?

What tests were done upon her arrival in the Emergency Department and why?

What was her reason for admission?

You should also click on **Diagnostic Reports** to learn what additional tests or procedures were performed and when. Finally, review the **Nursing Admission** and **History and Physical** to learn about the health history of this patient. When you are done reviewing the chart, click **Return to Nurses' Station**.

MEDICATIONS

Open the Medication Administration Record (MAR) by clicking on the **MAR** icon in the tool bar at the top of your screen. *Remember:* The MAR automatically opens to the first occupied room number on the floor—which is not necessarily your patient's room number! Since you need to access Dorothy Grant's MAR, click on tab **201** (her room number). Always make sure you are giving the *Right Drug to the Right Patient!*

Examine the list of medications ordered for Dorothy Grant. In the table below, list the medications that need to be given during this period of care (0730-0815). For each medication, note the dosage, route, and time to be given.

Time	Medication	Dosage	Route

Click on **Return to Nurses' Station**. Next, click on **201** on the bottom tool bar and then verify that you are indeed in Dorothy Grant's room. Select **Clinical Alerts** (the icon to the right of Initial Observations) to check for any emerging data that might affect your medication administration priorities. Next, go to the patient's chart (click on the **Chart** icon; then click on **201**). When the chart opens, select the **Physician's Orders** tab.

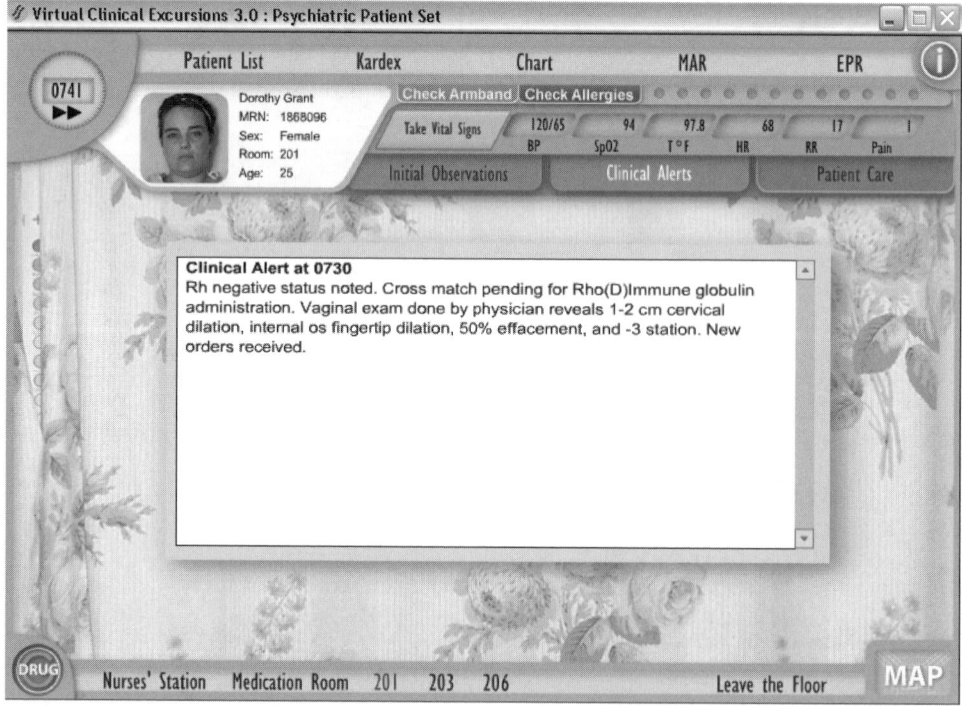

Review the orders. Have any new medications been ordered? Return to the MAR (click **Return to Room 201**; then click **MAR**). Verify that any new medications have been correctly transcribed to the MAR. Mistakes are sometimes made in the transcription process in the hospital setting, and it is sound practice to double-check any new order.

Are there any patient assessments you will need to perform before administering these medications? If so, return to Room 201 and click on **Patient Care** and then **Physical Assessment** to complete those assessments before proceeding.

Now click on the **Medication Room** icon in the tool bar at the bottom of your screen to locate and prepare the medications for Dorothy Grant.

In the Medication Room, you must access the medications for Dorothy Grant from the specific dispensing system in which each medication is stored. Locate each medication that needs to be given in this time period and click on **Put Medication on Tray** as appropriate. (*Hint:* Look in **Unit Dosage** drawer first.) When you are finished, click on **Close Drawer** and then on **View Medication Room**. Now click on the medication tray on the counter on the left side of the medication room screen to begin preparing the medications you have selected. (*Remember:* You can also click **Preparation** in the tool bar at the top of the screen.)

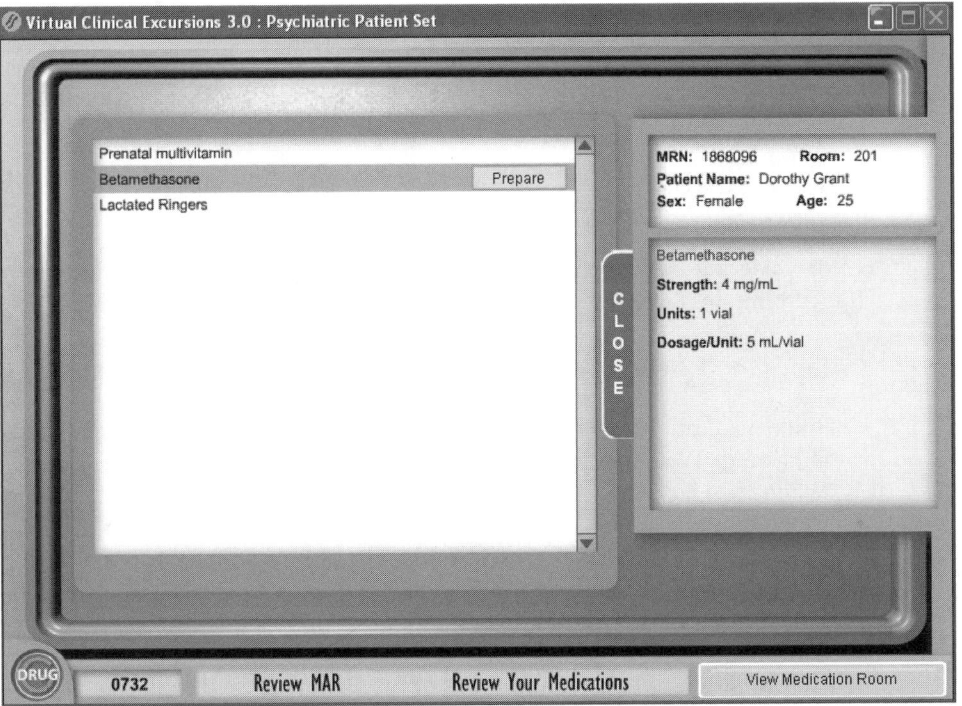

In the preparation area, you should see a list of the medications you put on the tray in the previous steps. Click on the first medication and then click **Prepare**. Follow the onscreen instructions of the Preparation Wizard, providing any data requested. As an example, let's follow the preparation process for betamethasone, one of the medications due to be administered to Dorothy Grant during this period of care. To begin, click to select **Betamethasone**; then click **Prepare**. Now work through the Preparation Wizard sequence as detailed below:

Amount of medication in the ampule: Betamethasone 5 mL.
Enter the amount of medication you will draw up into a syringe: **3 mL**.
Click **Next**.
Select the patient to receive the medication: **Room 201, Dorothy Grant**.
Click **Finish**.
Click **Return to Medication Room**.

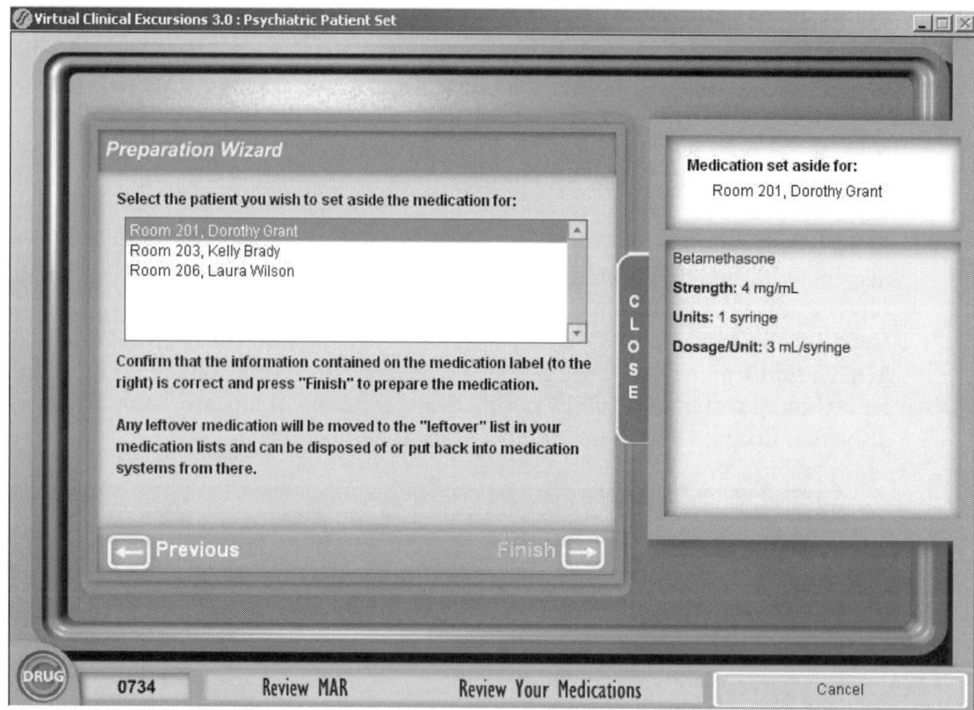

Follow this same basic process for the other medications due to be administered to Dorothy Grant during this period of care. (*Hint:* Look in **IV Storage** and **Automated System**.)

PREPARATION WIZARD EXCEPTIONS

- Some medications in *Virtual Clinical Excursions—Psychiatric* are prepared by the pharmacy (e.g., IV antibiotics) and taken to the patient room as a whole. This is common practice in most hospitals.
- Blood products are not administered by students through the *Virtual Clinical Excursions—Psychiatric* simulations since blood administration follows specific protocols not covered in this program.
- The *Virtual Clinical Excursions—Psychiatric* simulations do not allow for mixing more than one type of medication, such as regular and Lente insulins, in the same syringe. In the clinical setting, when multiple types of insulin are ordered for a patient, the regular insulin is drawn up first, followed by the longer-acting insulin. Insulin is always administered in a special unit-marked syringe.

Now return to Room 201 (click on **201** on the bottom tool bar) to administer Dorothy Grant's medications.

At any time during the medication administration process, you can perform a further review of systems, take vital signs, check information contained within the chart, or verify patient identity and allergies. Inside Dorothy Grant's room, click **Take Vital Signs**. (*Note:* These findings change over time to reflect the temporal changes you would find in a patient similar to Dorothy Grant.)

When you have gathered all the data you need, click on **Patient Care** and then select **Medication Administration**. Any medications you prepared in the previous steps should be listed on the left side of your screen. Let's continue the administration process with the betamethasone ordered for Dorothy Grant. Click to highlight **Betamethasone** in the list of medications. Next, click on the down arrow to the right of **Select** and choose **Administer** from the drop-down menu. This will activate the Administration Wizard. Complete the Wizard sequence as follows:

- Route: **Injection**
- Method: **Intramuscular**
- Site: **Any** (choose one)
- Click **Administer to Patient** arrow.
- Would you like to document this administration in the MAR? **Yes**
- Click **Finish** arrow.

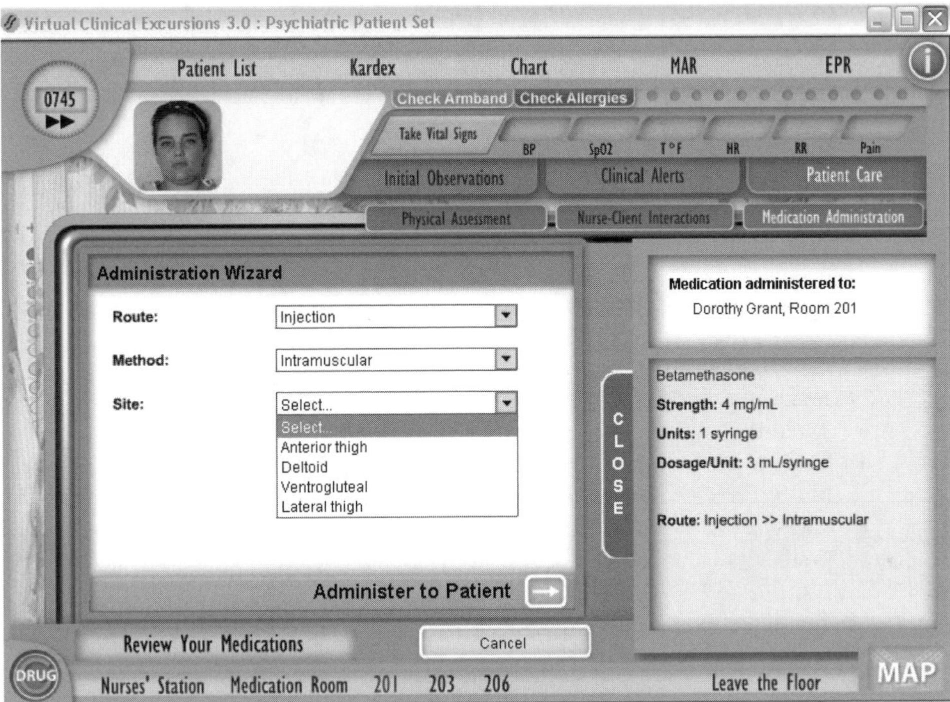

Your selections are recorded by a tracking system and evaluated on a Medication Scorecard stored under Preceptor's Evaluations. This scorecard can be viewed, printed, and given to your instructor. To access the Preceptor's Evaluations, click on **Leave the Floor**. When the Floor Menu appears, select **Look at Your Preceptor's Evaluation**. Then click on **Medication Scorecard** inside the box with Dorothy Grant's name (see example on the following page).

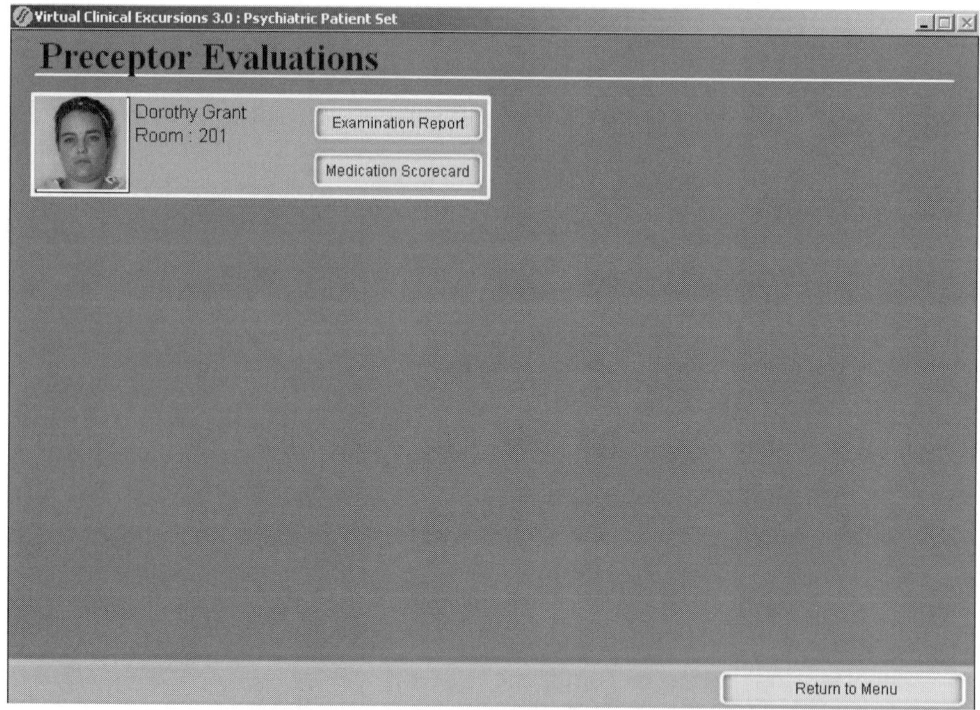

MEDICATION SCORECARD

- First, review Table A. Was betamethasone given correctly? Did you give the other medications as ordered?
- Table B shows you which (if any) medications you gave incorrectly.
- Table C addresses the resources used for Dorothy Grant. Did you access the patient's chart, MAR, EPR, or Kardex as needed to make safe medication administration decisions?
- Did you check the patient's armband to verify her identity? Did you check whether your patient had any known allergies to medications? Were vital signs taken?

When you have finished reviewing the scorecard, click **Return to Evaluations** and then **Return to Menu**.

■ VITAL SIGNS

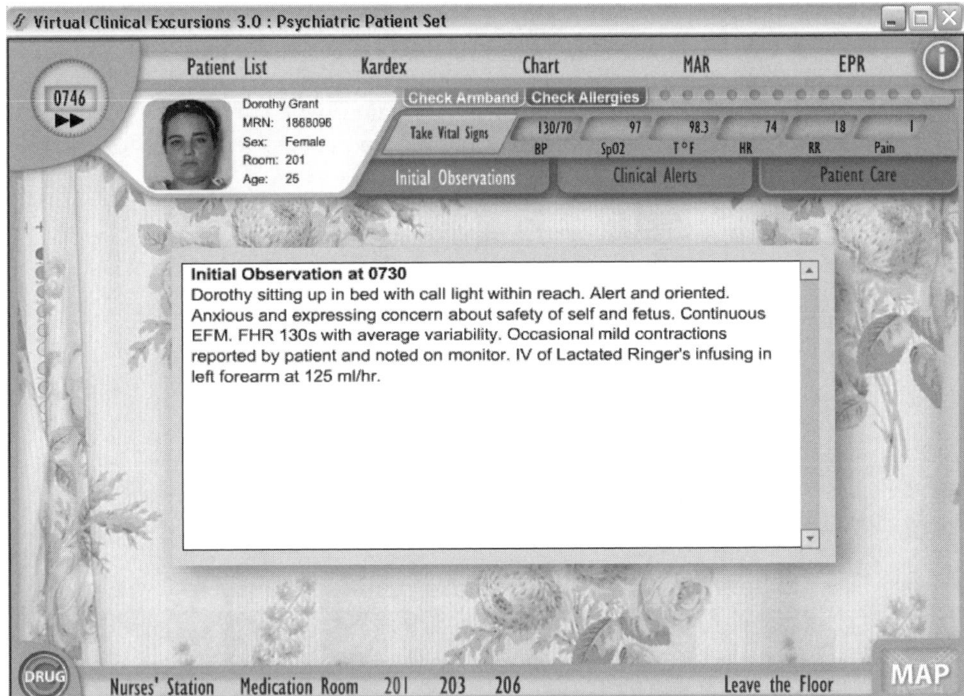

Vital signs, often considered the traditional "signs of life," include body temperature, heart rate, respiratory rate, blood pressure, oxygen saturation of the blood, and pain level.

Inside Dorothy Grant's room, click **Take Vital Signs**. (*Note:* If you are following this detailed tour step by step, you will need to **Restart the Program** from the Floor Menu, sign in again, and navigate to Room 201.) Collect vital signs for this patient and record them for Period of Care 1 below. Note the time at which you collected each of these data. (*Remember:* You can take vital signs at any time. The data change over time to reflect the temporal changes you would find in a patient similar to Dorothy Grant.)

Vital Signs	Findings/Time
Blood pressure	
O_2 saturation	
Temperature	
Heart rate	
Respiratory rate	
Pain rating	

After you are done, click on the **EPR** icon located in the tool bar at the top of the screen. Your username and password are automatically provided. Click on **Login** to enter the EPR. To access Dorothy Grant's records, click on the down arrow next to Patient and choose her room number, **201**. Select **Vital Signs** as the category. Next, in the empty time column on the far right, record the vital signs data you just collected in Dorothy Grant's room. (*Note:* If you need help with this process, see page 16.) Now compare these findings with the data you collected earlier for this patient's vital signs. Use these earlier findings to establish a baseline for each of the vital signs.

a. Are any of the data you collected significantly different from the baseline for a particular vital sign?

Circle One: Yes No

b. If "Yes," which data are different?

PHYSICAL ASSESSMENT

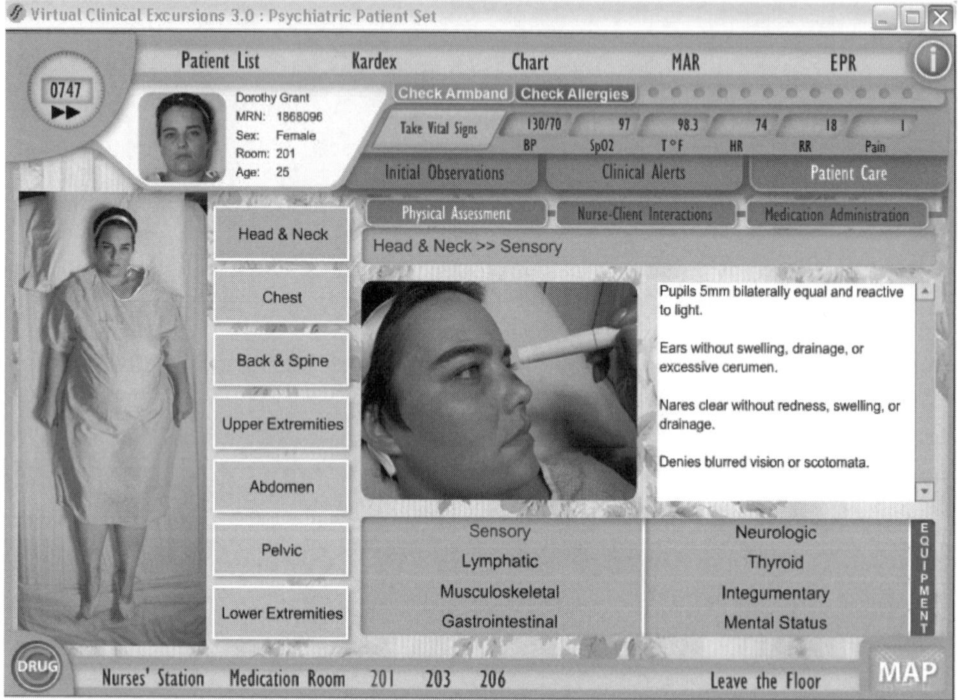

After you have finished examining the EPR for vital signs, click **Exit EPR** to return to Room 201. Click **Patient Care** and then **Physical Assessment**. Think about any information you received in the report at the beginning of this shift, as well as what you may have learned about this patient from the chart. Based on this, what area(s) of examination should you pay most attention to at this time? Is there any equipment you should be monitoring? Conduct a physical assessment of the body areas and systems that you consider priorities for Dorothy Grant. For example, select **Head & Neck**; then click on and assess **Sensory** and **Lymphatic**. Complete any other assessment(s) you think are necessary at this time. In the following table, record the data you collected during this examination.

Area of Examination	Findings
Head & Neck Sensory	
Head & Neck Lymphatic	

After you have finished collecting these data, return to the EPR. Compare the data that were already in the record with those you just collected.

a. Are any of the data you collected significantly different from the baselines for this patient?

   Circle One: Yes No

b. If "Yes," which data are different?

NURSE-CLIENT INTERACTIONS

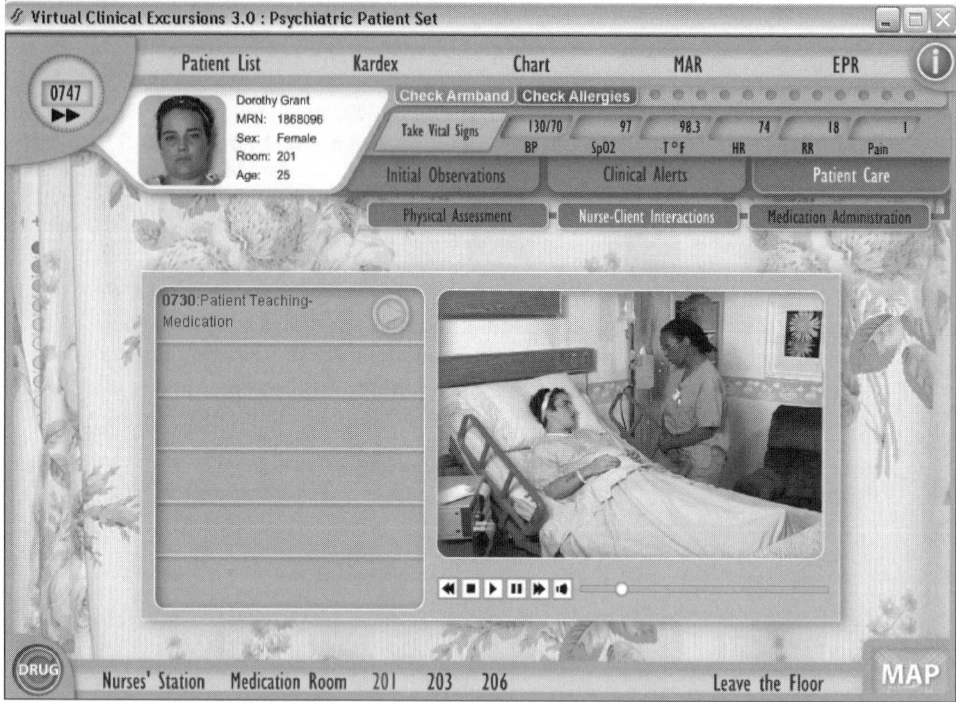

Click on **Patient Care** from inside Dorothy Grant's room (201). Now click on **Nurse-Client Interactions** to access a short video titled **Patient Teaching—Medication**, which is available for viewing at or after 0730 (based on the virtual clock in the upper left corner of your screen; see *Note* below). To begin the video, click on the white arrow next to its title. You will observe a nurse communicating with Dorothy Grant. There are many variations of nursing practice, some exemplifying "best" practice and some not. Note whether the nurse in this interaction displays professional behavior and compassionate care. Are her words congruent with what is going on with the patient? Does this interaction "feel right" to you? If not, how would you handle this situation differently? Explain.

Note: If the video you wish to view is not listed, this means you have not yet reached the correct virtual time to view that video. Check the virtual clock; you may return to access the video once its designated time has occurred—as long as you do so within the same period of care. Or you can click on the fast-forward icon within the virtual clock to advance the time by 2-minute intervals. You will then need to click again on **Patient Care** and **Nurse-Client Interactions** to refresh the screen.

At least one Nurse-Client Interactions video is available during each period of care. Viewing these videos can help you learn more about what is occurring with a patient at a certain time and also prompt you to discern between nurse communications that are ideal and those that need improvement. Compassionate care and the ability to communicate clearly are essential components of delivering quality nursing care, and it is during your clinical time that you will begin to refine these skills.

COLLECTING AND EVALUATING DATA

Each of the activities you perform in the Patient Care environment generates a significant amount of assessment data. Remember that after you collect data, you can record your findings in the EPR. You can also review the EPR, patient's chart, videos, and MAR at any time. You will get plenty of practice collecting and then evaluating data in context of the patient's course.

Now, here's an important question for you:

> Did the previous sequence of exercises provide the most efficient way to assess Dorothy Grant?

For example, you went to the patient's room to get vital signs, then back to the EPR to enter data and compare your findings with extant data. Next, you went back to the patient's room to do a physical examination, then again back to the EPR to enter and review data. If this back-and-forth process of data collection and recording seemed inefficient, remember the following:

- Plan all of your nursing activities to maximize efficiency, while at the same time optimizing the quality of patient care. (Think about what data you might need before performing certain tasks. For example, do you need to check a heart rate before administering a cardiac medication or check an IV site before starting an infusion?)
- You collect a tremendous amount of data when you work with a patient. Very few people can accurately remember all these data for more than a few minutes. Develop efficient assessment skills, and record data as soon as possible after collecting them.
- Assessment data are only the starting point for the nursing process.

Make a clear distinction between these first exercises and how you actually provide nursing care. These initial exercises were designed to involve you actively in the use of different software components. This workbook focuses on sensible practices for implementing the nursing process in ways that ensure the highest-quality care of patients.

Most important, remember that a human being changes through time, and that these changes include both the physical and psychosocial facets of a person as a living organism. Think about this for a moment. Some patients may change physically in a very short time (a patient with emerging myocardial infarction) or more slowly (a patient with a chronic illness). Patients' overall physical and psychosocial conditions may improve or deteriorate. They may have effective coping skills and familial support, or they may feel alone and full of despair. In fact, each individual is a complex mix of physical and psychosocial elements, and at least some of these elements usually change through time.

Thus it is crucial that you *DO NOT* think of the nursing process as a simple one-time, five-step procedure consisting of assessment, nursing diagnosis, planning, implementation, and evaluation. Rather, the nursing process should be utilized as a creative and systematic approach to delivering nursing care. Furthermore, because all living organisms are constantly changing, we must apply the nursing process over and over. Each time we follow the nursing process for an individual patient, we refine our understanding of that patient's physical and psychosocial conditions based on collection and analysis of many different types of data. *Virtual Clinical Excursions—Psychiatric* will help you develop both the creativity and the systematic approach needed to become a nurse who is equipped to deliver the highest-quality care to all patients.

REDUCING MEDICATION ERRORS

Earlier in this detailed tour, you learned the basic steps of medication preparation and administration. The following simulations will allow you to practice those skills further—with an increased emphasis on reducing medication errors by using the Medication Scorecard to evaluate your work.

Sign in to work on the Obstetrics Floor at Pacific View Regional Hospital for Period of Care 1. (*Note:* If you are already working with another patient or during another period of care, click on **Leave the Floor** and then **Restart the Program**; then sign in.)

From the Patient List, select Dorothy Grant. Then click on **Go to Nurses' Station**. Complete the following steps to prepare and administer medications to Dorothy Grant.

- Click on **Medication Room** on the tool bar at the bottom of your screen.
- Click on **MAR** and then on tab **201** to determine prn medications that have been ordered for Dorothy Grant. (*Note:* You may click on **Review MAR** at any time to verify the correct medication orders. Always remember to check the patient name on the MAR to make sure you have the correct patient's record. You must click on the correct room number tab within the MAR.) Click on **Return to Medication Room** after reviewing the correct MAR.
- Click on **Unit Dosage** (or on the Unit Dosage cabinet); from the close-up view, click on drawer **201**.
- Select the medications you would like to administer. After each selection, click **Put Medication on Tray**. When you are finished selecting medications, click **Close Drawer** and then **View Medication Room**.
- Click on **Automated System** (or on the Automated System unit itself). Click **Login**.
- On the next screen, specify the correct patient and drawer location.
- Select the medication you would like to administer and click **Put Medication on Tray**. Repeat this process if you wish to administer other medications from the Automated System.
- When you are finished, click **Close Drawer** and **View Medication Room**.
- From the Medication Room, click **Preparation** (or on the preparation tray).
- From the list of medications on your tray, highlight the correct medication to administer and click **Prepare**.
- This activates the Preparation Wizard. Supply any requested information; then click **Next**.
- Now select the correct patient to receive this medication and click **Finish**.
- Repeat the previous three steps until all medications that you want to administer are prepared.
- You can click **Review Your Medications** and then **Return to Medication Room** when ready. Once you are back in the Medication Room, go directly to Dorothy Grant's room by clicking on **201** at the bottom of the screen.
- Inside the patient's room, administer the medication, utilizing the six rights of medication administration. After you have collected the appropriate assessment data and are ready for administration, click **Patient Care** and then **Medication Administration**. Verify that the correct patient and medication(s) appear in the left-hand window. Highlight the first medication you wish to administer; then click the down arrow next to Select. From the drop-down menu, select **Administer** and complete the Administration Wizard by providing any information requested. When the Wizard stops asking for information, click **Administer to Patient**. Specify **Yes** when asked whether this administration should be recorded in the MAR. Finally, click **Finish**.

SELF-EVALUATION

Now let's see how you did during your medication administration!

- Click on **Leave the Floor** at the bottom of your screen. From the Floor Menu, select **Look at Your Preceptor's Evaluation**. Then click on **Medication Scorecard**.

The following exercises will help you identify medication errors, investigate possible reasons for these errors, and reduce or prevent medication errors in the future.

1. Start by examining Table A. These are the medications you should have given to Dorothy Grant during this period of care. If each of the medications in Table A has a ✓ by it, then you made no errors. Congratulations!

If any medication has an X by it, then you made one or more medication errors.

Compare Tables A and B to determine which of the following types of errors you made: Wrong Dose, Wrong Route/Method/Site, or Wrong Time. Follow these steps:

a. Find medications in Table A that were given incorrectly.
b. Now see if those same medications are in Table B, which shows what you actually administered to Dorothy Grant.
c. Comparing Tables A and B, match the Strength, Dose, Route/Method/Site, and Time for each medication you administered incorrectly.
d. Then, using the form below, list the medications given incorrectly and mark the errors you made for each medication.

Medication	Strength	Dosage	Route	Method	Site	Time
	❑	❑	❑	❑	❑	❑
	❑	❑	❑	❑	❑	❑
	❑	❑	❑	❑	❑	❑
	❑	❑	❑	❑	❑	❑

2. To help you reduce future medication errors, consider the following list of possible reasons for errors.

- Did not check drug against MAR for correct medication, correct dose, correct patient, correct route, correct time, correct documentation.
- Did not check drug dose against MAR three times.
- Did not open the unit dose package in the patient's room.
- Did not correctly identify the patient using two identifiers.
- Did not administer the drug on time.
- Did not verify patient allergies.
- Did not check the patient's current condition or vital sign parameters.
- Did not consider why the patient would be receiving this drug.
- Did not question why the drug was in the patient's drawer.
- Did not check the physician's order and/or check with the pharmacist when there was a question about the drug or dose.
- Did not verify that no adverse effects had occurred from a previous dose.

Based on the list of possibilities you just reviewed, determine how you made each error and record the reason in the form below:

Medication	Reason for Error

3. Look again at Table B. Are there medications listed that are not in Table A? If so, you gave a medication to Dorothy Grant that she should not have received. Complete the following exercises to help you understand how such an error might have been made.

   a. Perhaps you gave a medication that was on Dorothy Grant's MAR for this period of care, without recognizing that a change had occurred in the patient's condition, which should have caused you to reconsider. Review patient records as necessary and complete the following form:

Medication	Possible Reasons Not to Give This Medication

   b. Another possibility is that you gave Dorothy Grant a medication that should have been given at a different time. Check her MAR and complete the form below to determine whether you made a Wrong Time error:

Medication	Given to Dorothy Grant at What Time	Should Have Been Given at What Time

c. Maybe you gave another patient's medication to Dorothy Grant. In this case, you made a Wrong Patient error. Check the MARs of other patients and use the form below to determine whether you made this type of error:

Medication	Given to Dorothy Grant	Should Have Been Given to

4. The Medication Scorecard provides some other interesting sources of information. For example, if there is a medication selected for Dorothy Grant but it was not given to her, there will be an X by that medication in Table A, but it will not appear in Table B. In that case, you might have given this medication to some other patient, which is another type of Wrong Patient error. To investigate further, look at Table D, which lists the medications you gave to other patients. See whether you can find any medications ordered for Dorothy Grant that were given to another patient by mistake. However, before you make any decisions, be sure to cross-check the MAR for other patients because the same medication may have been ordered for multiple patients. Use the following form to record your findings:

Medication	Should Have Been Given to Dorothy Grant	Given by Mistake to

5. Now take some time to review the medication exercises you just completed. Use the form below to create an overall analysis of what you have learned. Once again, record each of the medication errors you made, including the type of each error. Then, for each error you made, indicate specifically what you would do differently to prevent this type of error from occurring again.

Medication	Type of Error	Error Prevention Tactic

Submit this form to your instructor if required as a graded assignment, or simply use these exercises to improve your understanding of medication errors and how to reduce them.

Name: ______________________________ Date: ____________________

The following icons are used throughout this workbook to help you quickly identify particular activities and assignments:

 Indicates a reading assignment—tells you which textbook chapter(s) you should read before starting each lesson

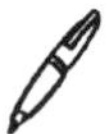 Indicates a writing activity

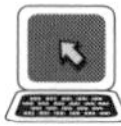 Marks the beginning of an interactive virtual hospital activity—signals you to open or return to your *Virtual Clinical Excursions—Psychiatric* simulation

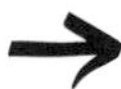 Indicates additional virtual hospital instructions

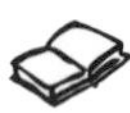 Indicates questions and activities that require you to consult your textbook

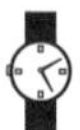 Indicates the approximate time required to complete an exercise

LESSON 1

Therapeutic Nurse-Patient Relationship

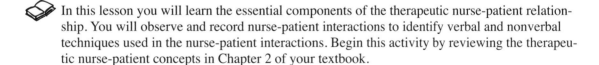

Reading Assignment: Therapeutic Nurse-Patient Relationship (Chapter 2)

Patients: Jacquline Catanazaro, Medical-Surgical Floor, Room 402
Kathryn Doyle, Skilled Nursing Floor, Room 503

Goal: To demonstrate an understanding of the importance of the therapeutic nurse-patient relationship and to identify and use therapeutic communication techniques with patients.

Objectives:

1. Understand the concept of the therapeutic nurse-patient relationship.
2. Identify the personal qualities of the nurse that are necessary to communicate effectively.
3. Define the phases of a therapeutic nurse-patient relationship.
4. Observe and identify effective communication techniques used by the nurse in nurse-patient interactions.
5. Discuss the concept of facilitative communication.
6. Discuss the importance of genuineness, respect, and empathy in the therapeutic nurse-patient relationship.
7. Understand types of therapeutic impasses in the nurse-patient relationship.
8. Identify motivational interviewing as an intervention for changing behaviors.

In this lesson you will learn the essential components of the therapeutic nurse-patient relationship. You will observe and record nurse-patient interactions to identify verbal and nonverbal techniques used in the nurse-patient interactions. Begin this activity by reviewing the therapeutic nurse-patient concepts in Chapter 2 of your textbook.

Exercise 1

Writing Activity

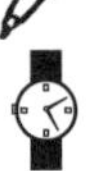

30 minutes

1. Define the therapeutic nurse-patient relationship.

2. The key therapeutic tool of the psychiatric nurse is the ______________________________.

3. There are six personal qualities the nurse must have in order to communicate therapeutically with patients. These are ___________________________________, ___________________________________, ___________________________________, ___________________________________, ___________________________________, and ___________________________________.

4. Identify the four phases of the nurse-patient relationship and the main task of each phase.

5. Discuss facilitative communication and its verbal and nonverbal components.

6. Discuss the qualities of genuineness, respect, and empathy that a nurse must have in order to establish and maintain a therapeutic relationship.

7. Describe how motivational interviewing assists patients to change their behavior.

8. Define therapeutic impass and discuss the four types of therapeutic impasses that can occur in a therapeutic relationship.

Exercise 2

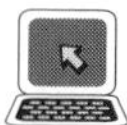

Virtual Hospital Activity

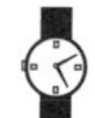

30 minutes

- Sign in to work at Pacific View Regional Hospital on the Medical-Surgical Floor for Period of Care 1. (*Note:* If you are already in the virtual hospital from a previous exercise, click on **Leave the Floor** and then on **Restart the Program** to get to the sign-in window.)
- From the Patient List, select Jacquline Catanazaro (Room 402).
- Click on **Get Report**.
- After reviewing the report, click on **Go to Nurses' Station**.
- Click on **402** at the bottom of the screen.
- Click on **Patient Care** and then on **Nurse-Client Interactions**.
- Select and view the video titled **0730: Intervention—Airway**. (*Note:* Check the virtual clock to see whether enough time has elapsed. You can use the fast-forward feature to advance the time by 2-minute intervals if the video is not yet available. Then click again on **Patient Care** and **Nurse-Client Interactions** to refresh the screen.)
- As you observe the nurse's verbal and nonverbal communication, complete the top row of the tables in questions 1 and 2.

Now let's jump ahead in virtual time to observe another interaction with this same patient.

- Click on **Leave the Floor**; then select **Restart the Program**.
- Sign in again for Jacquline Catanazaro, but this time choose Period of Care 2.
- Click on **Go to Nurses' Station**.
- Click on **402** to return to the patient's room.
- Click on **Patient Care** and then on **Nurse-Client Interactions**.
- Select and view the video titled **1115: Assessment—Readiness to Learn**. (*Note:* Check the virtual clock to see whether enough time has elapsed. You can use the fast-forward feature to advance the time by 2-minute intervals if the video is not yet available. Then click again on **Patient Care** and **Nurse-Client Interactions** to refresh the screen.)
- As you watch and listen to the video, complete the middle row of the tables in questions 1 and 2.

Now let's see how a nurse communicates with an older patient on the Skilled Nursing Floor.

- First, click on **Leave the Floor** and then on **Restart the Program**.
- This time, choose the Skilled Nursing Floor during Period of Care 1 and select Kathryn Doyle (Room 503) as your patient.
- Click on **Go to Nurses' Station**.
- Next, click on **503**, then on **Patient Care**, and then on **Nurse-Client Interactions**.
- Select and view the video titled **0730: Assessment—Biopsychosocial**. (*Note:* Check the virtual clock to see whether enough time has elapsed. You can use the fast-forward feature to advance the time by 2-minute intervals if the video is not yet available. Then click again on **Patient Care** and **Nurse-Client Interactions** to refresh the screen.)
- Use this video interaction to complete the bottom row in the tables in questions 1 and 2.

1. Based on the three videos you just viewed, complete the table below and on the next page by listing the therapeutic verbal communications used by the nurses. For each technique you list, identify the specific nurse communication you observed that demonstrates the technique.

Patient/POC	Verbal Therapeutic Communication Techniques Used by Nurse	Nurse Communication That Demonstrates Technique
Jacquline Catanazaro POC 1		
Jacquline Catanazaro POC 2		

Patient/POC	Verbal Therapeutic Communication Techniques Used by Nurse	Nurse Communication That Demonstrates Technique
Kathryn Doyle POC 1		

2. Based on the same three videos you used for question 1, document the nonverbal therapeutic communication techniques used by the nurses in the table below and on the next page.

Patient/POC	Type of Nonverbal Communication	Specific Nonverbal Therapeutic Techniques Used by the Nurse
Jacquline Catanazaro POC 1		

Patient/POC	Type of Nonverbal Communication	Specific Nonverbal Therapeutic Techniques Used by the Nurse
Jacquline Catanazaro POC 2		
Kathryn Doyle POC 1		

LESSON 2

The Stuart Stress Adaptation Model of Psychiatric Nursing Care

Reading Assignment: The Stuart Stress Adaptation Model of Psychiatric Nursing Care (Chapter 3)

Patient: Kelly Brady, Obstetrics Floor, Room 203

Goal: To care for a patient with both medical and psychiatric illnesses using the Stuart Stress Adaptation Model.

Objectives:

1. Identify the biopsychosocial components of care using the Stuart Stress Adaptation Model.
2. Use the Stuart Stress Adaptation Model to assess patients.
3. Participate in the care of an obstetric patient who has a comorbid psychiatric disorder.
4. Identify the predisposing and precipitating stressors of the patient.
5. Evaluate the significance of the patient's stressors.
6. Determine the patient's coping resources and coping mechanisms.
7. Identify the patient's stage of treatment and implement corresponding nursing interventions.

Exercise 1

Virtual Hospital Activity

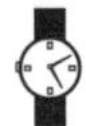

45 minutes

- Sign in to work at Pacific View Regional Hospital on the Obstetrics Floor for Period of Care 3. (*Note:* If you are already in the virtual hospital from a previous exercise, click on **Leave the Floor** and then on **Restart the Program** to get to the sign-in window.)
- From the Patient List, select Kelly Brady (Room 203).
- Click on **Get Report**. Review the report; then click on **Go to Nurses' Station**.
- Click on **Chart** and then on **203**.
- Click on the **Nursing Admission**.

1. What did you read in Kelly Brady's history that indicates she has had mental health problems in the past?

2. Let's consider precipitating stressors. What are three recent stressful life events that might contribute to Kelly Brady's depression and anxiety?

3. What is Kelly Brady's affective response to her depression?
   a. Cries often and does not want to be alone
   b. Does not show her sadness
   c. Rocks back and forth
   d. Talks with friends

4. According to the Nursing Admission, what is Kelly Brady's main coping mechanism?

5. How does Kelly Brady feel about her hospitalization?

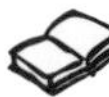

As you continue caring for Kelly Brady, use the information you have read in her chart and the change-of-shift report. You may also refer to pages 52-55 of your textbook.

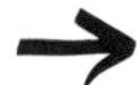

- Click on **Return to Nurses' Station**.
- Click on **203** at the bottom of the screen.
- Click on **Patient Care** and then on **Nurse-Client Interactions**.
- Select and view the video titled **1500: Transfer to Labor and Delivery**. (*Note:* Check the virtual clock to see whether enough time has elapsed. You can use the fast-forward feature to advance the time by 2-minute intervals if the video is not yet available. Then click again on **Patient Care** and **Nurse-Client Interactions** to refresh the screen.)

6. Considering the final aspect of the Stuart Stress Adaptation Model, what is Kelly Brady's treatment stage?
   a. Crisis
   b. Acute
   c. Maintenance
   d. Health Promotion

7. Given Kelly Brady's stage of treatment, answer the questions below to identify the nurse's goal, assessment, interventions, and expected outcomes. For each of these components, identify the nurse's action in the video that illustrates your answer.

   a. What is the overall nursing goal? What action illustrates this?

   b. What should the nurse assessment focus on? What action illustrates this?

   c. What is the purpose of the nurse's intervention? What action illustrates this?

   d. What is the expected outcome? What action illustrates this?

LESSON 3

The Biopsychosocial, Cultural, and Spiritual Context of Nursing Care

Reading Assignment: Biological Context of Psychiatric Nursing Care (Chapter 5)
Psychological Context of Psychiatric Nursing Care (Chapter 6)
Social, Cultural, and Spiritual Context of Psychiatric Nursing Care (Chapter 7)

Patient: Carlos Reyes, Skilled Nursing Floor, Room 504

Goal: To be able to discuss the biopsychosocial, cultural, and spiritual aspects of nursing care.

Objectives:

1. Understand normal structure and function of the brain.
2. Define neurotransmission as it relates to brain function and psychiatric disorders.
3. Understand the function and content of the mental status examination to determine mental-health functioning.
4. Understand the role that culture plays in the diagnosis and treatment of mental illness.
5. Understand the risk factors associated with age, gender, education, and income in relation to mental health and/or illness.

Exercise 1

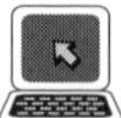

Virtual Hospital Activity

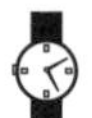

45 minutes

- Sign in to work at Pacific View Regional Hospital on the Skilled Nursing Floor for Period of Care 1. (*Note:* If you are already in the virtual hospital from a previous exercise, click on **Leave the Floor** and then on **Restart the Program** to get to the sign-in window.)
- From the Patient List, select Carlos Reyes (Room 504).
- Click on **Get Report** and review the report.
- Click on **Go to Nurses' Station**.
- Click on **Chart** and then on **504**.
- Read the **History and Physical** and **Nursing Admission** sections.

1. According to the History and Physical and the Nursing Admission, Carlos Reyes has two psychiatric diagnoses: ________________________________ and ________________.

2. Match each part of the brain to its function as it relates to Carlos Reyes' diagnoses.

	Part of the Brain	Function
_____	Limbic system	a. Learning, abstracting, reasoning
_____	Temporal lobe	b. Attention, emotions, memory
_____	Frontal lobe	c. Verbal and speech behaviors

→
- Click on **Return to Nurses' Station**.
- Click on **504** at the bottom of the screen.
- Click on **Patient Care** and then on **Physical Assessment**.
- From the body system categories (yellow buttons) select **Head & Neck**.
- From the subcategories (green buttons) select **Mental Status**.

3. The mental status report reveals which of the following important findings?
   a. Oriented to person and place only
   b. Sluggish speech patterns
   c. Impaired short-term memory
   d. High anxiety and agitation
   e. Choices a, b, and c only

4. Two biological factors affecting Carlos Reyes' brain function that need to be considered in caring for him are ____ and

   ____.

5. Define cultural competence and discuss its importance as a psychiatric nursing skill.

6. Discuss the biopsychosocial, cultural, and spiritual factors that must be considered in caring for Carlos Reyes.

→ • Still in the patient's room, click on **Nurse-Client Interactions**.

- Select and view the video titled **0740: Family Teaching—Medication**. (*Note:* Check the virtual clock to see whether enough time has elapsed. You can use the fast-forward feature to advance the time by 2-minute intervals if the video is not yet available. Then click again on **Patient Care** and **Nurse-Client Interactions** to refresh the screen.)
- Now click on the **Drug** icon in the lower left corner. Using either the Search box or the scroll bar at the top of the screen, find and select the entry for **oxazepam**.

7. Identify the indication(s) for oxazepam and the effect it has on brain function. What side effect was concerning Carlos Reyes' son during the video?

→ • Now, select and view the video titled **0745: Drowsiness—Contributing Factor**. (*Note:* Check the virtual clock to see whether enough time has elapsed. You can use the fast-forward feature to advance the time by 2-minute intervals if the video is not yet available. Then click again on **Patient Care** and **Nurse-Client Interactions** to refresh the screen.)

8. Two interventions the nurse used to answer Carlos Reyes' son's concerns regarding his father's drowsiness were ____ and ____.

9. What other actions could the nurse have taken?

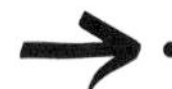

- Finally, select and view the video titled **0750: Assessment—Level of Assistance**. (*Note:* Check the virtual clock to see whether enough time has elapsed. You can use the fast-forward feature to advance the time by 2-minute intervals if the video is not yet available. Then click again on **Patient Care** and **Nurse-Client Interactions** to refresh the screen.)

10. What aspects of the mental status examination is the nurse attempting to assess?
    a. Appearance, speech, motor activity, and interaction
    b. Level of consciousness
    c. Emotional state: mood and affect
    d. All of the above

11. Assess the level of assistance Carlos Reyes needs in order to sit up and eat his breakfast.

LESSON 4

Families as Resources, Caregivers, and Collaborators

Reading Assignment: Families as Resources, Caregivers, and Collaborators (Chapter 10)

Patient: Jacquline Catanazaro, Medical-Surgical Floor, Room 402

Goal: To understand the role of the family in caring for a patient with mental illness.

Objectives:

1. Identify the characteristics of functional families.
2. Learn the benefits of partnering with the families of patients with mental illness.
3. Describe the focus of the competence model in working with the patient's family.
4. Identify barriers involved in educating families.
5. List one community advocacy group that can help families of the mentally ill.

Exercise 1

Writing Activity

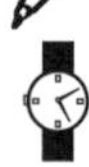

45 minutes

1. The ten elements of a functional family are listed below and on the next two pages. Briefly describe or explain each element as it specifically applies to the healthy, functional family.

Elements of a Functional Family	Qualities
1. Life cycle tasks	
2. Handling conflict	
3. Emotional contact	
4. Boundaries	

Elements of a Functional Family	Qualities
5. Problem solving	
6. Differences	
7. Children	
8. Emotional climate	
9. Balance	

Elements of a Functional Family	Qualities
10. Communication	

2. Partnering with ____________________ is an essential part of nursing care.

3. List at least two benefits of partnering with the families of patients with mental illness.

4. The competence model of care focuses on ______________________,

______________________, ______________________, ______________________, and

______________________ instead of dependency.

5. Describe a best practice intervention that is helpful to families of patients with mental illness.

6. List four barriers the nurse might experience when involving families in treatment.

7. Name one community advocacy group that could be helpful to families of the mentally ill patient.

Exercise 2

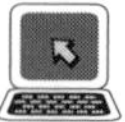

Virtual Hospital Activity

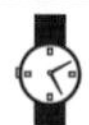

30 minutes

- Sign in to work at Pacific View Regional Hospital on the Medical-Surgical Floor for Period of Care 2. (*Note:* If you are already in the virtual hospital from a previous exercise, click on **Leave the Floor** and then on **Restart the Program** to get to the sign-in window.)
- From the Patient List, select Jacquline Catanazaro (Room 402).
- Click on **Go to Nurses' Station**.
- Click on **Chart** and then on **402**.
- Review the **Nursing Admission** and **History and Physical** sections of the chart.

1. What family information would be helpful to know before working with Jacquline Catanazaro's family?

2. A complete family history usually includes:
   a. information about all family members across three generations.
   b. the use of a genogram to organize the information.
   c. the health status of all members.
   d. current household living arrangements.
   e. relationships among the members.
   f. all of the above.

3. Discuss why you think it is important for the nurse to provide patient teaching regarding Jacquline Catanazaro's medication with her sister present.

4. What are two issues the sister will most likely have to deal with after Jacquline Catanazaro is discharged?

5. What type of psychoeducational assistance would be helpful to Jacquline Catanazaro's sister?
   a. Education about mental illness and community resources
   b. Practical approaches to help cope with symptomatic behavior
   c. Reinforcing of family strengths
   d. Allowing family members to share their concerns
   e. All of the above

LESSON 5

Crisis Intervention

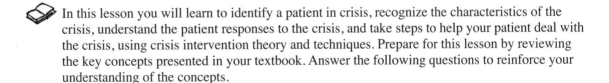

Reading Assignment: Crisis and Disaster Intervention (Chapter 13)

Patient: Dorothy Grant, Obstetrics Floor, Room 201

Goal: To understand how to provide nursing care for a patient in a health crisis using crisis intervention theory and techniques.

Objectives:

1. Define the characteristics and types of crises.
2. Describe the phases of a response to a crisis.
3. Understand two types of crises.
4. Define crisis and crisis intervention.
5. Discuss the cultural factors related to crisis intervention.
6. Understand the steps in crisis intervention.
7. Gain knowledge of techniques used to deal with patients in crisis.

In this lesson you will learn to identify a patient in crisis, recognize the characteristics of the crisis, understand the patient responses to the crisis, and take steps to help your patient deal with the crisis, using crisis intervention theory and techniques. Prepare for this lesson by reviewing the key concepts presented in your textbook. Answer the following questions to reinforce your understanding of the concepts.

Exercise 1

Writing Activity

30 minutes

1. A ____________________ is a disturbance caused by a stressful event or a perceived threat.

2. Describe the three phases a person may go through in a response to a crisis.

3. The three balancing factors present in a crisis that help an individual see the crisis realistically, support the individual in solving the problem, and offer effective coping are

   ______________________________________, ______________________________________,

   and ______________________________________.

4. Describe two types of crises and give an example of each.

5. ______________________________ is a brief, focused, and time-limited (approximately 6 weeks in length) treatment strategy that has been shown to be effective in helping people cope with stressful events in their lives. The goal of crisis intervention is to help the individual ____.

6. Describe how culture can play a crucial role in crisis intervention.

7. Explain the steps the nurse would take in providing crisis intervention and list the corresponding crisis intervention components within each step.

Crisis Intervention Steps	Crisis Intervention Components
Assessment	
Planning and implementation	
Evaluation	

8. Match each crisis intervention technique with its explanation.

	Technique	Explanation
_____	Catharsis	a. Nurse helps the patient to regain feelings of self-worth.
_____	Clarification	b. Nurse reinforces healthy behavior.
_____	Suggestion	c. Nurse promotes the release of feelings by the patient.
_____	Reinforcement of behavior	d. Nurse and patient actively explore solutions to the crisis.
_____	Support of defenses	e. Nurse helps the patient identify the relationship among the events, behaviors, and feelings.
_____	Raising self-esteem	f. Nurse encourages the use of healthy defenses and discourages those that are maladaptive.
_____	Exploration of solutions	g. Nurse influences the patient to accept an idea or belief.

Exercise 2

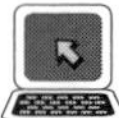

Virtual Hospital Activity

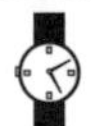

30 minutes

- Sign in to work at Pacific View Regional Hospital on the Obstetrics Floor for Period of Care 1. (*Note:* If you are already in the virtual hospital from a previous exercise, click on **Leave the Floor** and then on **Restart the Program** to get to the sign-in window.)
- From the Patient List, select Dorothy Grant (Room 201).
- Click on **Get Report**.

1. What information in the shift report would alert the nurse that a more thorough psychosocial assessment is needed?

It is important for the nurse to obtain more complete information to properly care for Dorothy Grant.

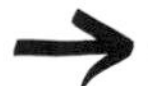

- Click on **Go to Nurses' Station**.
- Click on **Chart** and then on **201**.
- Access and review the **History and Physical** and **Nursing Admission** sections.

2. In the History and Physical, what information specifically indicates that Dorothy Grant may be in crisis?
   a. Dorothy Grant is 30 weeks pregnant.
   b. Her husband beat her and kicked her in the abdomen.
   c. Her children are at home alone.
   d. Her mother was beaten by her father.

3. The first step in crisis intervention is assessing the patient in five important areas. Based on your review of the Nursing Admission, what assessment information did the nurse obtain in each of the following areas regarding Dorothy Grant's abuse by her husband?

Elements of Crisis Intervention Assessment	Assessment Data Found
Precipitating event	
Perception of the event by the patient	
Support system of the patient	
Coping resources of the patient	
Coping mechanisms of the patient	

4. Given Dorothy Grant's perception of the event and her coping mechanisms, what crisis intervention techniques might work best at this time?

5. Provide one example of how the nurse could help Dorothy Grant regain her self-worth.

LESSON 6

Prevention, Mental Health Promotion, and Recovery Support in the Hospital and Community

Reading Assignment: Prevention and Mental Health Promotion (Chapter 12)
Recovery Support (Chapter 14)
Hospital-Based Psychiatric Nursing Care (Chapter 33)
Community-Based Psychiatric Nursing Care (Chapter 34)

Patient: Harry George, Medical-Surgical Floor, Room 401

Goal: To understand the role of the nurse in mental health prevention and promotion in the continuum of care for a complex patient across treatment settings.

Objectives:

1. Understand the goals of mental health promotion and prevention.
2. Discuss strategies used by the nurse in mental health prevention.
3. Describe the levels of mental health prevention.
4. Discuss the differences between the rehabilitation and recovery models.
5. Understand the steps involved in assessing a patient's need for recovery.
6. Discuss the community's influence on mental health recovery.
7. Understand the role of the nurse in caring for a complex patient with both chronic medical and mental health problems.
8. Discuss evidenced-based community treatment interventions that help patients with substance abuse disorders.

In this lesson you will learn about the role of the nurse in the continuum of care from mental health promotion and illness prevention to hospitalization and aftercare treatment options in the community.

Exercise 1

Writing Activity

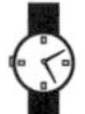

30 minutes

1. Match each prevention model with its description.

	Prevention Model	Definition
_____	Public health	a. Promotes mental health and prevention of mental illness by focusing on risk factors, vulnerability, and human response. The "patient" may be the individual, the family, or the community.
_____	Medical	b. The "patient" is the community, so the emphasis is on reducing the risk for mental illness for an entire population by providing services to the high-risk group.
_____	Nursing	c. Focuses on biological and brain research to discover specific causes of mental illness in the individual patient.

2. Match each prevention planning strategy with its intended purpose.

	Planning Strategy	Purpose
_____	Health education	a. Strengthens supports to increase their protective factor
_____	Environmental change	b. Dispels myths and stereotypes associated with vulnerable populations
_____	Social support	c. Helps to strengthen confidence in the patient
_____	Stigma reduction	d. Focuses on modification of the person's social/living situation to increase nurturing and positive reinforcement for the individual

3. Primary prevention activities in psychiatric nursing care have five basic aims. What are these goals?

4. Compare and contrast mental health recovery from mental health rehabilitation.

Model	Definition
Mental health recovery	
Mental health rehabilitation	

Nurses need to be aware of the range of patient care needs before, during, and after hospitalization.

5. In the public health model, tertiary prevention attempts to

 ____.

6. Name at least one agency or resource in your community that provides services to the mentally ill or to those with substance abuse disorders.

Exercise 2

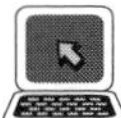

Virtual Hospital Activity

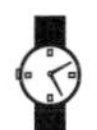

45 minutes

- Sign in to work at Pacific View Regional Hospital on the Medical-Surgical Floor for Period of Care 1. (*Note:* If you are already in the virtual hospital from a previous exercise, click on **Leave the Floor** and then on **Restart the Program** to get to the sign-in window.)
- From the Patient List, select Harry George (Room 401).
- Click on **Go to Nurses' Station**.
- Click on **Chart** and then on **401**.
- Click on and read the **History and Physical**.
- Click on and read the **Nursing Assessment**.

1. Based on the Nursing Prevention Model, which of the following stressors contributed to Harry George's current life situation?
   a. Motorcycle accident
   b. Chronic left foot bone infection and severe pain
   c. Estrangement from his wife and two sons
   d. Loss of job
   e. Homelessness
   f. All of the above

2. What stage of prevention activities would the nurse use during Harry George's stay in the hospital?
   a. Primary (health promotion)
   b. Secondary (crisis intervention)
   c. Tertiary (rehabilitation and recovery)

3. Match each type of health education intervention with the specific health topic Harry George will need to explore during hospitalization and after discharge.

	Type of Health Education Intervention	Specific Health Topic
_____	Increase awareness of issues related to health and illness	a. Developing healthy coping skills such as stress reduction; enhancing motivation and self-esteem; improving problem-solving and stress management skills
_____	Increase understanding of potential stressors, possible outcomes, and alternative coping responses	b. Learning how becoming clean and sober, caring for self, managing pain and diabetes, and smoking cessation can positively affect health
_____	Increase knowledge of where and how to obtain resources	c. Finding housing, finding/keeping job, and locating family members
_____	Increase actual abilities	d. Dealing with loss of family and job, homelessness, and pain

4. How important is pain management in Harry George's recovery? Explain.

5. In view of Harry George's current living situation and 4-year history of alcoholism, what do you think would be the best type of program to help him quit drinking after discharge?
   a. Community-based sober living house
   b. Inpatient alcohol/drug treatment program
   c. Outpatient visits with a drug/alcohol counselor
   d. Does not really matter since he will not stop drinking

6. What challenges does Harry George face in his recovery in the following areas of his life?

Area of Recovery	Challenge
Activities of daily living (ADL)	
Interpersonal relationships	

Area of Recovery	Challenge
Self-esteem	
Motivation	
Illness management	
Strengths	

7. What available hospital-based resources can the nurse use to help Harry George with the community needs he will have after discharge?

8. Using information from your textbook and taking into consideration Harry George's history and current needs, discuss how a positive change in his living/social environment could affect his recovery.

9. What are some possible community health services for which Harry George might be eligible?

LESSON 7

Patients with Anxiety Responses and Disorders

Reading Assignment: Anxiety Responses and Anxiety Disorders (Chapter 15)

Patient: Dorothy Grant, Obstetrics Floor, Room 201

Goal: To participate in the care of an obstetric patient who is experiencing anxiety.

Objectives:

1. Define anxiety and its essential features.
2. List the primary NANDA International nursing diagnoses associated with anxiety disorders.
3. Understand levels of anxiety.
4. Assess physiological responses to anxiety.
5. Discuss brain chemistry as it relates to anxiety.
6. Understand types of events leading to anxiety.
7. Discuss constructive and destructive reactions to anxiety.
8. Describe expected outcomes associated with anxiety.
9. Gain knowledge of medications prescribed for patients with anxiety.
10. Discuss levels of anxiety as they relate to nursing interventions.
11. Develop treatment interventions and expected outcomes for a patient with anxiety.

Exercise 1

Writing Activity

30 minutes

1. ____________________ is a vague sense of apprehension that includes feelings of uncertainty, helplessness, isolation, and insecurity.

2. The biological basis of anxiety involves three neurotransmitters in the brain. Explain the role each neurotransmitter plays in anxiety.

Neurotransmitter	Role in Anxiety
GABA	
Norepinephrine	
Serotonin	

3. Match each level of anxiety with its characteristics.

	Level	Characteristics
_____	Mild	a. Narrowing of the perceptual field as the person focuses on the immediate concerns
_____	Moderate	b. Associated with dread and terror; the personality becomes disorganized
_____	Severe	c. Associated with the tension of daily life
_____	Panic	d. Significant reduction in the perceptual field as the person focuses on details and cannot think of anything else

4. Identify at least two physiological responses to anxiety in each of the systems below and on the next page.

System	Physiological Responses
Cardiovascular	

System	Physiological Responses
Respiratory	
Gastrointestinal	
Neuromuscular	
Urinary tract	
Skin	

5. Match each type of response to anxiety with its group of characteristics.

	Type of Response	Characteristics
_____	Behavioral	a. Loss of objectiveness, poor concentration, preoccupation, thought blocking, decreased productivity
_____	Cognitive	b. Uneasiness, nervousness, impatience, jumpiness, fear, fright
_____	Affective	c. Rapid speech, restlessness, tremors, physical tension, hyperventilation

6. What are the four primary NANDA International nursing diagnoses concerned with anxiety responses?

7. Task-oriented reactions to anxiety are thoughtful, deliberate attempts to

    ________________________________, ________________________________, and

    ________________________________, whereas ego-oriented reactions, also

    called ________________________________, are often used to protect a person and are the first line of defense to successfully cope with mild to moderate anxiety.

8. Discuss three nursing interventions that are important when working with a patient with severe and panic levels of anxiety.

Exercise 2

Virtual Hospital Activity

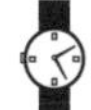

45 minutes

- Sign in to work at Pacific View Regional Hospital on the Obstetrics Floor for Period of Care 1. (*Note:* If you are already in the virtual hospital from a previous exercise, click on **Leave the Floor** and then on **Restart the Program** to get to the sign-in window.)
- From the Patient List, select Dorothy Grant (Room 201).
- Click on **Get Report**.

1. According to the change-of-shift report, what level of anxiety is Dorothy Grant experiencing?
   a. Mild
   b. Moderate
   c. Severe
   d. Panic

2. It is reported that Dorothy Grant's stated concerns of ______________________________

   and the ____ are causing her anxiety.

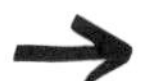

- Now click on **Go to Nurses' Station**.
- Click on **201** at the bottom of the screen.
- Click on **Patient Care** and then on **Nurse-Client Interactions**.
- Select and view the video titled **0730: Patient Teaching—Medication**. (*Note:* Check the virtual clock to see whether enough time has elapsed. You can use the fast-forward feature to advance the time by 2-minute intervals if the video is not yet available. Then click again on **Patient Care** and **Nurse-Client Interactions** to refresh the screen.)

3. How does the nurse's assessment of Dorothy Grant's anxiety level compare with the assessment described in the change-of-shift report?

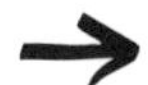

- Now click on **Chart** and then on **201**.
- Access and read the **Nursing Admission** section.

4. What are the two stressors listed that contribute to Dorothy Grant's anxiety?

5. Precipitating stressors can be grouped into two categories: threats to physical integrity and threats to self-system. How would you describe Dorothy Grant's stressors in terms of these two categories?

6. Dorothy Grant has been using maladaptive (destructive) coping mechanisms to handle her stressors. Next to each coping mechanism listed below, identify an alternative adaptive (constructive) mechanism.

Maladaptive (Destructive) Coping Mechanism	Adaptive (Constructive) Coping Mechanism
Hoping the abuse will stop	
Keeping the children quiet	
Blaming herself for causing the abuse (pregnancy)	
Trying not to upset her husband	

7. You have assessed Dorothy Grant's level of anxiety to be moderate in severity. Develop nursing interventions based on the following aspects of treatment.

Aspects	Nursing Interventions
Recognition	
Insight	
Education	
Coping	

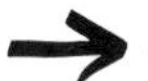

- Click on **Return to Room 201**.
- Click on **MAR** and review Dorothy Grant's medications.
- Check to see whether there are any medications ordered for Dorothy Grant's anxiety.

8. What classification of medications would be ordered for a patient with moderate to severe anxiety?
   a. Antidepressants
   b. Antianxiety agents
   c. Antipsychotics
   d. Stimulants

9. What are the key considerations in deciding whether to order medication to treat Dorothy Grant's anxiety? Select all that apply.

   _____ 30 weeks pregnant/possible contraindications

   _____ Anxiety initially assessed to be at a moderate level

   _____ Blunt force trauma to abdomen/may result in preterm delivery

   _____ Need more time to assess patient's anxiety

10. The best treatment outcomes will demonstrate adaptive ways of coping with stress. From the list below, choose two outcome statements that best describe desired outcomes based on Dorothy Grant's treatment plan.

    _____ Maintains adequate sleep

    _____ Plans coping strategies for stressful situations

    _____ Monitors behavioral manifestations of anxiety

    _____ Eliminates precursors of anxiety

LESSON 8

Patients with Emotional Responses and Mood Disorders

Reading Assignment: Emotional Responses and Mood Disorders (Chapter 18)

Patient: Kelly Brady, Obstetrics Floor, Room 203

Goal: To care for a patient who is experiencing a medical health crisis (severe preeclampsia at 26 weeks gestation) and also has symptoms of depression.

Objectives:

1. Understand depression in the context of the continuum of emotional responses.
2. Assess a patient who is demonstrating an unhealthy emotional state.
3. Identify behaviors associated with depression.
4. List the primary NANDA International nursing diagnoses associated with mood disorders.
5. Discuss the risk for suicide in patients with severe mood disturbance.
6. Understand the relationship between depressed mood and pregnancy.
7. Describe predisposing risk factors and precipitating stressors in depression.
8. Identify coping resources and mechanisms of patients with depression.
9. Describe effective interventions including pharmacological treatment for depressed patients.
10. Develop a treatment plan for a patient with depression.

Exercise 1

Writing Activity

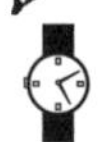

45 minutes

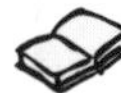

1. Using the continuum of emotional responses in your textbook, match each specific response with its corresponding type of response.

	Specific Response	Type of Response
_____	Emotional responsiveness	a. Adaptive
_____	Depression or mania	b. Maladaptive
_____	Suppression of emotions	
_____	Delayed grief reaction	
_____	Uncomplicated grief reaction	

2. Which of the following statements about depression is (are) true?
   a. 1 in 5 patients seen by a primary provider has significant symptoms of depression.
   b. Mood disturbances can be a specific response to stress.
   c. The lifetime risk for major depression in women is 20% to 30%.
   d. 85% of patients with depression can be treated successfully using a combination of verbal therapies and medication.
   e. Only one-third of all people with depression seek help, are accurately diagnosed, or are appropriately treated.
   f. Women of childbearing age face the highest demographic risk for depression.
   g. All of the above are true.

3. Complete the table below and on the next page by listing examples of symptoms associated with persons who have depression.

Type of Symptoms	Examples
Affective	

Type of Symptoms	Examples
Physiological	
Cognitive	
Behavioral	

4. What are the six primary NANDA International nursing diagnoses related to maladaptive emotional response?

5. People with depression have a genuine need to believe that things can get better. To help patients with this need, the nurse should do which of the following? Select all that apply.

_____ Express hope for the patient.

_____ Reinforce the fact that depression is a self-limiting disorder and the future will be better.

_____ Explain to the patient that depression is a chronic disease.

_____ Explain that expressing feelings is normal and necessary.

6. Evidence shows cognitive and behavioral interventions to be effective treatment for depression. The three objectives of cognitive strategies are

____,

____, and

____.

7. Successful behavior is a powerful tool to counteract depression. Discuss specific interventions the nurse can implement in caring for the depressed patient to effect positive behavioral change. Include three potentially rewarding activities that the patient can accomplish to make positive behavioral changes.

8. For treating patients with depression, which class of medications has proven the most effective with the least number of side effects?
   a. Selective serotonin reuptake inhibitors (SSRIs)
   b. Monoamine oxidase inhibitors (MAOIs)
   c. Tricyclic antidepressant drugs (TCAs)

9. How would the nurse educate the depressed patient on the importance of developing increased social skills?

10. List the four underlying principles that govern a psychoeducational program on depression for patients and their families.

Exercise 2

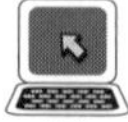

Virtual Hospital Activity

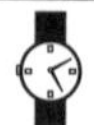

30 minutes

- Sign in to work at Pacific View Regional Hospital on the Obstetrics Floor for Period of Care 1. (*Note:* If you are already in the virtual hospital from a previous exercise, click on **Leave the Floor** and then on **Restart the Program** to get to the sign-in window.)
- From the Patient List, select Kelly Brady (Room 203).
- Click on **Get Report**. After reading the report, click on **Go to Nurses' Station**.
- Click on **203** at the bottom of the screen.
- Inside the patient's room, click on **Patient Care** and then on **Physical Assessment**.
- Click on **Head & Neck**.
- Click on **Mental Status**.

1. Based on the mental status assessment, Kelly Brady's two documented behavioral symptoms are ____________________ and ______________________________________.

- Now click on **Chart** and then on **203**.
- Click on and read the **History and Physical**.

2. Provide the following information based on your review of the patient's H&P.

   a. What is the predisposing factor in Kelly Brady's family history related to depression?

   b. What key fact related to depression did you find in her past medical history?

3. Kelly Brady had a diagnosed episode of depression in college. What percentage of those who have had depression in the past will eventually have it again?
   a. 10%
   b. 25%
   c. 50%
   d. 75%

- Still in the chart, click on **Mental Health** and read the Psychiatric Mental Health Assessment.
- Then click on **Consultations** and read the Psychiatric Consult.

4. According to the DSM-IV Axis I diagnosis and the patient's symptoms, where on the emotional response continuum does Kelly Brady fall?
   a. Emotional responsiveness
   b. Uncomplicated grief reaction
   c. Suppression of emotions
   d. Delayed grief reaction
   e. Depression

5. The continuum of emotional responses ranges from adaptive to maladaptive. The type of emotional response Kelly Brady is using is ________________________.

6. What major life events/precipitating stressor(s) is (are) contributing to Kelly Brady's mood disturbance?
   a. Lack of supports: mother has cancer, parents are out of town, and sister is going through divorce
   b. Financial stress: problems with her and her husband's jobs and moving into larger home
   c. Biological factors: pregnancy
   d. All of the above

7. List all the behavioral symptoms Kelly Brady is experiencing related to depression.

8. To begin developing a treatment plan to address Kelly Brady's depression, complete the intervention section of the treatment plan below.

Area	Goal	Intervention
Environment/safety	To keep patient safe	
Cognitive	To move patient beyond her preoccupation to other aspects of her life	
Behavioral	To accomplish tasks and activities to counteract depression	
Social skills	To provide experiences to counteract depression and social isolation and build self-esteem	
Education	To educate the patient about depression and identify the interventions and treatment that will be helpful	

9. Discuss how Kelly Brady's pregnancy might be related to her depression.

10. Kelly Brady's physician has recommended that she take paroxetine after the birth of her baby. Using what you have learned from the records you have read, fill in the blanks below.

 The trade name for paroxetine is ________________________, and the dose that was recommended was _______________. The clinical rationale for recommending paroxetine is that ____.

LESSON 9

Patients with Neurobiological Responses and Thought Disorders

Reading Assignment: Neurobiological Responses and Schizophrenia and Psychotic Disorders (Chapter 20)

Patient: Jacquline Catanazaro, Medical-Surgical Floor, Room 402

Goal: To care for a patient with chronic schizophrenia who is hospitalized for acute asthma.

Objectives:

1. Understand the range of neurobiological responses from adaptive to maladaptive and know where schizophrenia is located within the range.
2. List the positive and negative symptoms of schizophrenia.
3. Understand symptoms of schizophrenia in terms of their impact on the cognitive, perceptual, emotional, behavioral, and social aspects of the person's life.
4. Identify predisposing factors and precipitating stressors of schizophrenia and understand how to appraise stressors.
5. Identify coping resources the person with schizophrenia has available and recognize the coping mechanisms the person is using.
6. List the components of an education plan for a patient with schizophrenia.
7. Identify the components of discharge planning for a patient with schizophrenia.

Exercise 1

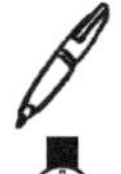

Writing Activity

15 minutes

1. psychosis refers to the mental state of not being in touch with reality.

   Schiazophrenia is a serious and persistent neurobiological brain disease that can severely impair the lives of individuals, their families, and communities.

2. In the continuum of neurobiological responses, schizophrenia would be considered a

   maladaptive response.

3. The impact of schizophrenia on the individual and society is enormous. Which of the following are true statements about schizophrenia? Select all that apply.

   X In the United States, about 2.5 million people suffer from schizophrenia (about 1 of every 100 Americans).

   _____ Of people diagnosed with schizophrenia, 100% have the disease for life.

   X In 75% of cases, the onset for schizophrenia is between the ages of 15 and 34.

   X 33% to 50% of homeless people in the United States have schizophrenia.

   _____ Individuals with schizophrenia have higher morbidity and mortality because of co-occurring medical illnesses.

   X 10% to 20% of patients with schizophrenia attempt suicide, and 5% succeed.

4. What is the overall goal of nursing care for a person with psychosis?

   To help the patient recognize symptoms and to manage them to help with recovery

5. It is important to understand and differentiate the positive and negative symptoms of schizophrenia. In the table below, identify the positive and negative symptoms associated with each category listed.

Category	Positive Symptoms	Negative Symptoms
Thinking	Delusions	Algia
Emotion		affective flattening
Speech	pressured speech	alogia
Behavior	bizzare behavior	apathy

6. Numerous stressors or triggers often precede a new episode or exacerbation of the symptoms of schizophrenia. Match each of the following triggers with its corresponding category.

	Common Relapse Trigger	Category of Stressor
C D	Low self-concept/self-confidence	a. Health
B	Lack of social support	b. Environment
B	Housing difficulties	c. Attitudes
D	Aggressive/violent behavior	d. Behavior
A	Lack of sleep	
C/D	Poor medication management	
B	Lack of transportation	
B	Financial problems	
C/D	Poor social skills	
A	Poor nutrition	
B	Social isolation	
A	Lack of exercise	

Exercise 2

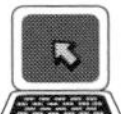

Virtual Hospital Activity

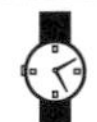

45 minutes

- Sign in to work at Pacific View Regional Hospital on the Medical-Surgical Floor for Period of Care 3. (*Note:* If you are already in the virtual hospital from a previous exercise, click on **Leave the Floor** and then on **Restart the Program** to get to the sign-in window.)
- From the Patient List, select Jacquline Catanazaro (Room 402).
- Click on **Go to Nurses' Station**.
- Click on **Chart** and then on **402**.
- Click on **Nurse's Notes**.
- Read the note written on admission on Monday at 1600.

1. Identify two pieces of information contained in the nurse's admission note that have implications for this patient's discharge planning.

 __X__ Patient has asthma.

 __X__ Sister is patient's main support.

 _____ Patient has no transportation.

 _____ Patient has a history of stopping her psychiatric medication.

→ • Now read the **Nurse's Notes** written on Tuesday at 0400.

2. Jacquline Catanazaro states that people are putting poison into her IV. This is an example of what type of delusion?
 a. Grandiose
 b. Persecutory
 (c.) Paranoid
 d. None of the above

→ • Now read the **Nurse's Notes** for Wednesday at 0600.

3. The note describes symptoms of schizophrenia that have a direct relationship to Jacquline Catanazaro's asthma. Explain the relationship.

 patient refuses nasal cannula because of suspicion of poison

→ • Now click on the **Consultation** tab in the chart.
• Read the Psychiatric Consult.

4. The positive symptom of schizophrenia described in the report is

Delusions, and the negative symptoms described are

affective flattening and

apathy.

5. The plan contained within the Psychiatric Consult includes exercise and nutrition. Comment on the relevance of diet and exercise as part of the plan of care for Jacquline Catanazaro.

execerise & nutrition can help

reduce needed drugs

→ • Click on and review the **History and Physical** and **Nursing Admission** sections.

6. For each category below, list Jacquline Catanazaro's barriers to compliance that may result in future relapses.

Category	Barriers to Compliance
Health	Shortness of breath
Thoughts	Delusions
Attitudes	Alexithymia
Behavior	negatism
Socialization	alone on disability
Medication	Stopped taking all meds

7. Education will be a critical component of Jacquline Catanazaro's treatment plan. From the list below, identify her educational needs. Select all that apply.

X Healthy living

X Medication

X Psychoeducation

X Illness management

→ • Click on **Return to Room 402**.
- Click on **MAR** and then on tab **402**.
- Scroll down to locate the antipsychotic medication ordered.
- Click on **Return to Room 402**.
- Click on the **Drug** icon in the lower left corner of the screen. Find the entry for this medication.

8. Based on your review of the Drug Guide, fill in the information requested below and on the next page.

Name of medication

ziprosidone

Indication

schizophrenia

Mechanism of action

Effects probably medicated by antagonism of dopamine type 2 + serotonin type 2

Side effects

nausea

Prolonged QT interval

Dosage

20 mg PO daily

Nursing considerations

Monitor mental status, mood, behavior, positive & negative symptoms

watch for severe reaction

Patient teaching

9. Review the medication dosage Jacquline Catanazaro is receiving and the usual dosage as stated in the Drug Guide. What might be the rationale for the current dosage the physician is giving to her?

Start at 20 mg

then may increase ~~by~~ q2 days

up to 80 mg q 12 hr

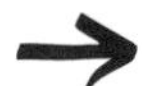

- Click on **Return to Room 402**.
- Click on **Patient Care** and then on **Nurse-Client Interactions**.
- Select and view the video titled **1500: Intervention—Patient Teaching**. (*Note:* Check the virtual clock to see whether enough time has elapsed. You can use the fast-forward feature to advance the time by 2-minute intervals if the video is not yet available. Then click again on **Patient Care** and **Nurse-Client Interactions** to refresh the screen.)
- After watching the 1500 video, select and view the video titled **1540: Discharge Planning**.

10. Discuss the importance of including Jacquline Catanazaro's sister in the discharge planning process.

support system &

help keep on medicine

LESSON 10

Patients with Cognitive Responses, Organic Mental Disorders, and Aggressive Behavior

Reading Assignment: Cognitive Responses and Organic Mental Disorders (Chapter 22)
Preventing and Managing Aggressive Behavior (Chapter 28)

Patient: Carlos Reyes, Skilled Nursing Floor, Room 504

Goal: To care for a patient who has symptoms of cardiovascular disease, cognitive impairment, and agitation.

Objectives:

1. Recognize the continuum of adaptive and maladaptive cognitive responses.
2. Compare and contrast definitions and characteristics of delirium and dementia.
3. Provide examples of severe disturbed behavior associated with dementia.
4. Identify structures in the brain responsible for aggressive behavior that often accompany maladaptive cognitive responses.
5. Identify precipitating stressors associated with delirium and dementia.
6. Discuss the high-priority nursing interventions in the treatment of patients with delirium and dementia.
7. Describe medications used in the treatment of dementia and agitation.
8. Identify underlying medical conditions that can produce symptoms of delirium.
9. Understand family involvement in discharge planning, including cultural aspects of care.

Exercise 1

Writing Activity

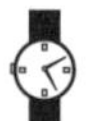

30 minutes

1. Maladaptive cognitive responses include which of the following? Select all that apply.

    _____ Inability to make decisions

    _____ Impaired memory and judgment

    _____ Oriented to person, time, and place

    _____ Misperceptions

    _____ Attention to detail

    _____ Difficulty with logical reasoning

2. Maladaptive cognitive responses are most apparent in people who have a diagnosis of
    a. delirium.
    b. dementia.
    c. both a and b.

3. Delirium is characterized by the ____________________ of awareness and a ____________________ onset, whereas dementia has a ____________________ onset and is characterized by the loss of ____________________ abilities of ____________________, ____________________, and ____________________.

4. In addition to the usual dementia symptoms of disorientation, confusion, memory loss, disorganized thinking, and poor judgment, some patients may experience more severe disturbed behavior. Below, match each category of behavior with its corresponding examples.

	Category of Behavior	**Examples of Behavior**
_____	Aggressive psychomotor behavior	a. Incontinence, poor hygiene
_____	Nonaggressive psychomotor behavior	b. Complaining, screaming, being disruptive and/or demanding
_____	Verbally aggressive behavior	c. Decreased activity, apathy, withdrawal
_____	Passive behavior	d. Hitting, kicking, pushing, scratching, assault
_____	Functionally impaired behavior	e. Restlessness, pacing, wandering

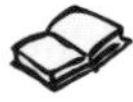

5. There are three structures in the brain implicated in aggressive behavior: the frontal lobe, limbic system, and hypothalamus. Below, describe the normal function of each area. Then identify signs and symptoms of dysfunction associated with each area. (See Chapter 28.)

Area of Brain	Function	Dysfunction
Frontal lobe		
Limbic system		
Hypothalamus		

6. Any major disruption in the balance of body functions can disrupt cognitive functioning. Discuss cardiac disorders and cardiac medications as potential precipitating stressors in delirium.

7. In caring for a patient experiencing symptoms of delirium, the nurse gives the highest priority to nursing interventions that ______________________________. Three nursing interventions that maintain life are ____, ____, and ____.

8. In providing care to patients with dementia, the nurse gives the highest priority to nursing interventions that maintain the patient's optimum level of functioning. Complete the table below and on the next page.

Component of Care	Interventions
Social interaction	
Medications	
Orientation	
Communication	

Component of Care	Interventions
Wandering	
Agitation	
Family and community	

Exercise 2

Virtual Hospital Activity

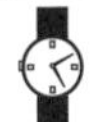

15 minutes

- Sign in to work at Pacific View Regional Hospital on the Skilled Nursing Floor for Period of Care 2. (*Note:* If you are already in the virtual hospital from a previous exercise, click on **Leave the Floor** and then on **Restart the Program** to get to the sign-in window.)
- From the Patient List, select Carlos Reyes (Room 504).
- Click on **Get Report**.
- Read both shift summaries in the report.

1. According to the shift reports, Carlos Reyes' most problematic symptoms have been

   ____,

   ____,

   and ____.

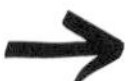

- Now click on **Go to Nurses' Station**.
- Click on **504** at the bottom of the screen.
- Click on **Patient Care**.
- Click on **Physical Assessment**.
- Click on **Head & Neck**.
- Click on and read **Mental Status**.

2. During the mental status assessment, what symptoms are described that indicate Carlos Reyes is having maladaptive cognitive responses?

3. Which of the following behaviors associated with aggression is Carlos Reyes exhibiting? Select all that apply.

_____ Extreme anxiety

_____ Irritability

_____ Soft-spoken voice

_____ Confusion

_____ Memory intact

_____ Disorientation

→ • Now click on **Nurse-Client Interactions**.

• Select and view the video titled **1120: The Agitated Patient**. (*Note:* Check the virtual clock to see whether enough time has elapsed. You can use the fast-forward feature to advance the time by 2-minute intervals if the video is not yet available. Then click again on **Patient Care** and **Nurse-Client Interactions** to refresh the screen.)

4. What intervention(s) did the nurse use to respond to Carlos Reyes' agitation? Select all that apply.

_____ Ignored the difficult behavior

_____ Listened to the patient and patient's daughter

_____ Spoke in a calm, reassuring manner to decrease stress in the environment

_____ Modified the original plan to meet the patient's needs

→ • Now select and view the video titled **1140: Assessing for Referrals**. (*Note:* Check the virtual clock to see whether enough time has elapsed. You can use the fast-forward feature to advance the time by 2-minute intervals if the video is not yet available. Then click again on **Patient Care** and **Nurse-Client Interactions** to refresh the screen.)

5. Assess Carlos Reyes' son's understanding of his father's illness. What action will the nurse need to take after her brief interaction with the son?

Exercise 3

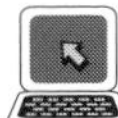

Virtual Hospital Activity

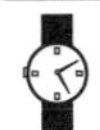

30 minutes

- Sign in to work at Pacific View Regional Hospital on the Skilled Nursing Floor for Period of Care 3. (*Note:* If you are already in the virtual hospital from a previous exercise, click on **Leave the Floor** and then on **Restart the Program** to get to the sign-in window.)
- From the Patient List, select Carlos Reyes (Room 504).
- Click on **Go to Nurses' Station**.
- Click on **Chart** and then on **504**.
- Read the **History and Physical** and **Nursing Admission**.

1. If Carlos Reyes returns to his daughter's home after discharge, discuss the problems that his daughter may have in caring for him.

2. Now that you have reviewed all the pertinent data, what factors may be contributing to Carlos Reyes' confusion? Select all that apply.

_____ Change in environment

_____ Recent myocardial infarction

_____ History of dementia

_____ Medication regime

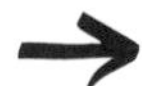

- Click on **Return to Nurses' Station**.
- Click on **504** to go to Carlos Reyes' room.
- Inside the room, click on **Patient Care** and then on **Nurse-Client Interactions**.
- Select and view the video titled **1500: The Confused Patient**. (*Note:* Check the virtual clock to see whether enough time has elapsed. You can use the fast-forward feature to advance the time by 2-minute intervals if the video is not yet available. Then click again on **Patient Care** and **Nurse-Client Interactions** to refresh the screen.)

3. Describe the approach the nurse used in dealing with Carlos Reyes' confusion.

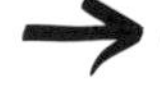

- Now select and view the video titled **1505: Family Teaching—Dementia**. (*Note:* Check the virtual clock to see whether enough time has elapsed. You can use the fast-forward feature to advance the time by 2-minute intervals if the video is not yet available. Then click again on **Patient Care** and **Nurse-Client Interactions** to refresh the screen.)

4. Describe the intervention the nurse used while interacting with Carlos Reyes.

- Click on **MAR** and select tab **504**.
- Review the medication ordered for Carlos Reyes' anxiety and agitation.
- Click on **Return to Room 504**.
- Click on the **Drug** icon in the lower left corner of the screen.
- Find and review this medication in the Drug Guide.

5. To identify the important aspects of this medication, provide the information requested below and on the next page.

Name of medication

Class

Mechanism of action

Therapeutic effect

Indication

Dosage

Side effects

Nursing indications

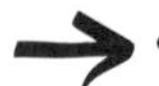

- Again click on **Return to Room 504**.
- Click on **Patient Care** and then on **Nurse-Client Interactions**.
- Select and view the video titled **1525: Family Conflict—Discharge Plan**. (*Note:* Check the virtual clock to see whether enough time has elapsed. You can use the fast-forward feature to advance the time by 2-minute intervals if the video is not yet available. Then click again on **Patient Care** and **Nurse-Client Interactions** to refresh the screen.)
- After observing the interaction, click on **Chart** and then on **504**.
- Click on **Consultations**.
- Read the Discharge Coordinator Consult.

6. Describe the family conflict associated with Carlos Reyes' care, its effect on discharge planning, and how the nurse should best approach the situation.

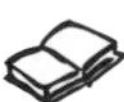

7. In successful discharge planning, practical recommendations are necessary for caregivers of patients with dementia, especially those who are also agitated and aggressive. Using your textbook and what you know about Carlos Reyes, provide some practical approaches below and on the next page that you believe would be helpful to his daughter, who is his sole caregiver.

Area of Focus	Practical Approaches
Decrease escalation	

Area of Focus	Practical Approaches
Communicate effectively	
Review the basics	

LESSON 11

Patients with Chemically Mediated Responses and Substance-Related Disorders

Reading Assignment: Chemically Mediated Responses and Substance-Related Disorders (Chapter 23)

Patient: Laura Wilson, Obstetrics Floor, Room 206

Goal: To care for a patient with acute medical needs who also has a diagnosis of polysubstance abuse.

Objectives:

1. Recognize the continuum of adaptive and maladaptive chemically mediated responses.
2. Understand behaviors of abuse and dependence.
3. Describe predisposing factors, precipitating stressors, and appraisal of stressors related to substance abuse.
4. Examine the nurse's own feelings about working with a patient who is pregnant and HIV-positive and has polysubstance abuse.
5. Identify nursing diagnosis as it relates to polysubstance abuse.
6. Identify key aspects of a treatment plan that includes patient teaching for a patient with polysubstance abuse.
7. Discuss issues involved in discharge planning of a patient who has polysubstance abuse.

Exercise 1

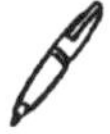

Writing Activity

15 minutes

1. Drugs that affect the pleasure centers of the brain and therefore create pleasurable changes in the mental and emotional states have the greatest potential for abuse. Alcohol and cocaine are very popular because they produce effects on the brain within minutes.

2. Identify the potential drugs of abuse in the following list. Select all that apply.

   X Alcohol

   X Cocaine

   ____ Marijuana

   X Prescription pain medications

   X Heroin

   X Inhalants

   ____ Prescription diet pills

   ____ Prescription antianxiety medications

3. Not everyone who uses drugs becomes an abuser; however, for some users, the range of chemically mediated coping responses begins with adaptive responses and progresses to Maladaptive responses and eventually leads to abuse and dependence.

4. An understanding of the terminology related to abuse is important when discussing chemically mediated coping responses. Match each term with its corresponding definition.

	Term	Definition
C	Substance abuse	a. The psychosocial behaviors related to substance dependence
D	Substance dependence	b. Occurs when there is a coexistence of substance abuse and a psychiatric disorder
A	Addiction	c. Continued use of substances despite related problems
B	Dual diagnosis	d. Severe condition (usually considered a disease) that may include physical problems and serious disruption in the person's life
E	Withdrawal symptoms	e. Caused by a biological need that occurs when the body becomes used to having the substance in the system
F	Tolerance	f. Occurs with continued use, as more of the substance is needed to produce the same effect

5. Discuss the importance of testing for the presence of drugs in patients who present with possible substance abuse.

very prevalent + substance disorders are under diagnosed

6. Lifestyles associated with substance abuse carry risks. Which of the following lifestyle risks are associated with substance abuse? Select all that apply.

X Accidents

X Violence

X Self-neglect

X Physical and mental illnesses

X Complications during pregnancy

X Fetal abnormalities and substance dependence

X Hepatitis B and C

X HIV and AIDS

7. In terms of the predisposing factors of substance abuse, several models have been proposed within the biological, psychological, and sociocultural spheres. Since a belief in a particular model influences the way in which the nurse thinks about and will work with the patient, discuss your beliefs about persons with substance abuse.

I think that they made the decision to start and that it's their own problem

Exercise 2

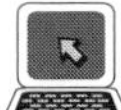

Virtual Hospital Activity

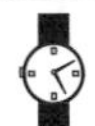

15 minutes

- Sign in to work at Pacific View Regional Hospital on the Obstetrics Floor for Period of Care 1. (*Note:* If you are already in the virtual hospital from a previous exercise, click on **Leave the Floor** and then on **Restart the Program** to get to the sign-in window.)
- From the Patient List, select Laura Wilson (Room 206).
- Click on **Get Report**.
- After reading the report, click on **Go to Nurses' Station**.
- Click on **Chart** and then on **206**.
- Click on **Emergency Department** and read the report.

1. What information alerts the nurse that Laura Wilson may be abusing drugs? Select all that apply.

   __X__ Found unconscious

   _____ Nausea and diarrhea

   __X__ HIV-positive status

   __X__ History of drug abuse

2. Laura Wilson's urine drug screen came back positive for marijuana and cocaine. Complete the table below and on the next page regarding the characteristics of these two drugs.

Substance	Route	Signs and Symptoms of Use	Withdrawal Signs and Symptoms	Consequences of Use
Cocaine	Snorting injection	restlessness pananoid irritability anxiety	depression fatigue mood changes agitation	Stroke G I ~~bleer~~ ulcers

Substance	Route	Signs and Symptoms of Use	Withdrawal Signs and Symptoms	Consequences of Use
Marijuana	Smoke	Rapid HR Increased BP Increased RR Red eyes Dry mouth Increased appetite Slow reaction time	Aggression Anxiety Depressed mood Decreased appetite	rapid HR disorientation lack of physical coodination ~~often~~ depression sleepiness panic attacks anxiety

- Still in the chart, click on **Nursing Admission**.
- Read the report.

3. In addition to caffeine, Laura Wilson is abusing two other drugs. According to the Nursing Admission, these two drugs are Cocaine and Marijuana.

4. Explain how these drugs might affect the health of her baby.

defects

baby may go through withdraw

MR

underweight

5. The Nursing Admission record contains information regarding Laura Wilson's precipitating stressors. Which of the following stressors has Laura Wilson identified? Select all that apply.

X Parents' disapproval of her lifestyle

X HIV-positive status

X Unplanned pregnancy

X Desire to quit "crack"

X Boyfriend out of town

6. Select the best coping resource that might be available to Laura Wilson.
   a. Younger sister
   b. Boyfriend
   c. Mother and father
   d. Roommate

7. Laura Wilson's most frequently used coping mechanisms for dealing with her problems are denile and anxiety.

Exercise 3

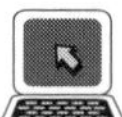

Virtual Hospital Activity

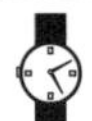

30 minutes

- Sign in to work at Pacific View Regional Hospital on the Obstetrics Floor for Period of Care 2. (*Note:* If you are already in the virtual hospital from a previous exercise, click on **Leave the Floor** and then on **Restart the Program** to get to the sign-in window.)
- From the Patient List, select Laura Wilson (Room 206).
- Click on **Get Report**.
- After reading the report, click on **Go to Nurses' Station**.
- Click on **206** at the bottom of the screen.
- Click on **Patient Care** and then on **Nurse-Client Interactions**.
- Select and view the video titled **1115: Teaching—Effects of Drug Use**. (*Note:* Check the virtual clock to see whether enough time has elapsed. You can use the fast-forward feature to advance the time by 2-minute intervals if the video is not yet available. Then click again on **Patient Care** and **Nurse-Client Interactions** to refresh the screen.)

1. Which of the following statements made by Laura Wilson illustrates her lack of understanding regarding substance abuse? Select all that apply.

   X "The baby will help me stay on track."

   X "It's not like I'm addicted. I can quit anytime."

   X "It's not like the baby will be addicted."

2. Which of the following statements made by the patient may indicate her readiness to abstain from drugs? Select all that apply.

   X "It wasn't a hard decision for me. I am looking forward to this baby."

   _____ "I can go for a while without taking drugs."

   X "My mom doesn't believe I can do it."

   X "I'll do whatever it takes to keep my baby."

3. What potential barriers can you identify that may interfere with Laura Wilson's abstinence from drugs?

   She thinks occasional use is OK.

4. Evaluate the nurse's role in educating Laura Wilson on the effects of drug use.

its very important because she has many misconceptions

→ • Click on **MAR**.
• Find the medication ordered for Laura Wilson's pain.
• Click on **Return to Room 206**.
• Click on the **Drug** icon in the lower left corner of the screen.
• Locate and review the entry for this medication.

5. The medication ordered for Laura Wilson's pain is Fentanyl Citrate. Given her medical condition, the two most important features of this medication are that it is safe to use in pregnancy and it is not harmful.

6. An important aspect of Laura Wilson's treatment will be the teaching plan. Match each of her education needs with the intervention that will best help her with that need.

	Education Need	Effective Intervention
C	HIV-positive status	a. Well-baby clinic and parental support
A	Caring for her newborn	b. Community AA-based self-help group and individual motivational and cognitive behavioral approaches
D	Drug abstinence	c. HIV counselor/HIV clinic
E	Handling family conflict	d. Consultation with hospital social worker/ discharge planner
B	Community resources	e. Family counseling

7. For patients who abuse substances, a key aspect of discharge planning is a relapse prevention plan, developed together by the nurse and patient. Discuss the key elements of the relapse prevention plan for Laura Wilson.

Baby's safety /need

own safety

provide knowledge for disease substance abuse

promote social group

LESSON 12

Patients with Eating Regulation Responses and Eating Disorders

Reading Assignment: Eating Regulation Responses and Eating Disorders (Chapter 24)

Patient: Tiffany Sheldon, Pediatrics Floor, Room 305

Goal: To provide nursing care for a patient with an eating disorder who also has comorbid psychiatric symptoms.

Objectives:

1. Identify behaviors associated with eating disorders.
2. Describe the continuum of adaptive and maladaptive eating disorder regulation responses.
3. Discuss predisposing factors and precipitating stressors related to eating disorders.
4. Assess interactions between the nurse and a patient with an eating disorder.
5. Identify coping resources and coping mechanisms related to eating disorders.
6. Assess and plan care for a patient with an eating disorder.
7. Identify the psychological components of a treatment plan for a patient with an eating disorder.
8. Identify desired outcomes for a patient with an eating disorder.

Exercise 1

Writing Activity

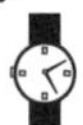

15 minutes

1. Food is essential to life but can also be used to satisfy unmet ____________________ needs, to moderate ____________________, and to provide ____________________ and ____________________.

2. Which of the following symptoms and/or behaviors best reflect maladaptive eating regulation response? Select all that apply.

    _____ Night eating syndrome

    _____ Skipping meals occasionally

    _____ Anorexia

    _____ Severe dieting

    _____ Overeating under stress

    _____ Bulimia

    _____ Frequent fasting

    _____ Binge eating disorder

3. The psychological reasons for disordered eating can lead to serious biological changes such as ________________________, ____, and ________________________. Psychological problems associated with eating disorders include ________________________, ________________________, and ________________________.

4. How do sociocultural factors regarding body size affect the prevalence of eating disorders?

5. Many factors may predispose a person to develop an eating disorder. Which of the following psychological factors would be associated with eating disorders? Select all that apply.

_____ Rigid, meticulous, and ritualistic personality or behavioral traits

_____ No early childhood issues

_____ Pervasive sense of ineffectiveness and helplessness

_____ Understanding the feelings of others

_____ Difficulty tolerating intense emotional states

_____ Fear of biological or psychological maturity

6. Many people who are in treatment for eating disorders show evidence of other psychiatric disorders. For each type of eating disorder listed below, identify the possible psychiatric comorbidity.

Eating Disorder	Psychiatric Comorbidity
Anorexia	
Bulimia	
Anorexia and bulimia	
Binge eating disorder	
Night eating disorder	

7. Discuss the environmental factors that may predispose someone to an eating disorder.

8. What feelings do you have regarding patients who have eating disorders that result in being severely underweight or overweight? How might sociocultural factors play a part in these feelings? Do you recognize any personal bias toward patients with these problems? Explain.

Exercise 2

Virtual Hospital Activity

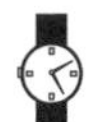

15 minutes

- Sign in to work at Pacific View Regional Hospital on the Pediatrics Floor for Period of Care 1. (*Note:* If you are already in the virtual hospital from a previous exercise, click on **Leave the Floor** and then on **Restart the Program** to get to the sign-in window.)
- From the Patient List, select Tiffany Sheldon (Room 305).
- Click on **Get Report**.

1. Based on the shift report, the possible psychiatric behaviors Tiffany Sheldon is exhibiting

   are ____, ______________________, and

   ______________________.

- Click on **Go to Nurses' Station**.
- Click on **305** at the bottom of the screen.
- Click on **Patient Care** and then on **Physical Assessment**.
- Click on **Head & Neck** and then on **Mental Status**.

2. Based on the shift report and the findings of the mental status assessment, identify the characteristics that apply to Tiffany Sheldon. Select all that apply.

   _____ Good eye contact

   _____ Listlessness

   _____ Flat affect

   _____ Energetic

   _____ Avoids eye contact

   _____ Withdrawn

- Click on **Nurse-Client Interactions**.
- Select and view the video titled **0730: Initial Assessment**. (*Note:* Check the virtual clock to see whether enough time has elapsed. You can use the fast-forward feature to advance the time by 2-minute intervals if the video is not yet available. Then click again on **Patient Care** and **Nurse-Client Interactions** to refresh the screen.)

3. Describe your reaction to Tiffany Sheldon's responses to the nurse who is caring for her.

→ • Click on **Chart** and then on **305**.
• Click on **Physician's Orders**.

4. Which orders indicate that multidimensional assessments (in addition to physical assessments) are being implemented for Tiffany's care? Select all that apply.

_____ Nursing supervision during and after meals

_____ Nutritionist to follow patient

_____ Involvement of adolescent care team

_____ Involvement of eating disorders clinic

_____ Consultation with psychiatric team

→ • Click on **History and Physical** and review.

5. Tiffany Sheldon's medical diagnoses are ________________________,

________________________, and ________________________.

→ • Click on **Nursing Admission** and review.

6. List at least two possible psychological and two environmental predisposing factors associated with Tiffany's eating disorder.

Exercise 3

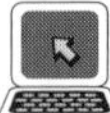

Virtual Hospital Activity

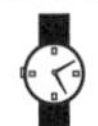

30 minutes

- Sign in to work at Pacific View Regional Hospital on the Pediatrics Floor for Period of Care 3. (*Note:* If you are already in the virtual hospital from a previous exercise, click on **Leave the Floor** and then on **Restart the Program** to get to the sign-in window.)
- From the Patient List, select Tiffany Sheldon (Room 305).
- Click on **Get Report** and review the report.
- Click on **Go to Nurses' Station**.
- Click on **305** at the bottom of the screen.
- Click on **Patient Care** and then on **Nurse-Client Interactions**.
- Select and view the video titled **1500: Relapse—Contributing Factors**. (*Note:* Check the virtual clock to see whether enough time has elapsed. You can use the fast-forward feature to advance the time by 2-minute intervals if the video is not yet available. Then click again on **Patient Care** and **Nurse-Client Interactions** to refresh the screen.)

1. Tiffany's predisposing factors make her especially vulnerable to environmental pressures and stress. Identify the stressors that have contributed to her current relapse of her eating disorder. Select all that apply.

   _____ Parents divorced 3 years ago.

   _____ Family does not understand her problem.

   _____ Mom is angry and "disgusted."

   _____ Visited her father in Florida 2 weeks ago.

→ • Click on **Chart** and then on **305**.
- Click on **Mental Health**.
- Read the Psychiatric Assessment.

2. Characteristic of those who have anorexia, Tiffany's main maladaptive coping mechanism

   is ________________________.

3. For people with anorexia, the issue is not really about their weight, but rather about controlling life and fears. Tiffany's statement, "____," is an example of this overriding concern.

4. In addition to Tiffany Sheldon's nursing diagnosis of Imbalanced nutrition less than body requirements, identify two nursing diagnoses that best describe the psychological components to her eating disorder.

- Click on **Return to Room 305**.
- Click on **Patient Care** and then on **Nurse-Client Interactions**.
- Select and view the video titled **1530: Facilitating Success**. (*Note:* Check the virtual clock to see whether enough time has elapsed. You can use the fast-forward feature to advance the time by 2-minute intervals if the video is not yet available. Then click again on **Patient Care** and **Nurse-Client Interactions** to refresh the screen.)

5. One of the most important parts of assessing a patient with an eating disorder is determining the person's motivation to change the behavior. What statement does Tiffany make that best defines her motivation level and has implications for her success in preventing relapse?

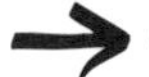

- Click on **Chart** and then on **305**.
- Click on **Consultations**.
- Read the Psychiatric Consult.

6. Two plans of care are being implemented simultaneously for Tiffany Sheldon. One plan involves the eating contract. The other is the plan devised as a result of the Psychiatric Consult. Complete the table below and on the next page by describing elements of the plan outlined in the Psychiatric Consult.

Psychosocial Treatment Plan	Specific interventions
Individual therapy	
Family conference/family therapy	

Relationship to eating contract

Medication

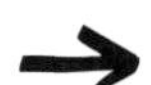

- Still in the chart, click on **Patient Education**.
- Read the report.

7. Identify the expected treatment outcomes for Tiffany. Can you think of other important outcomes?

LESSON 13

Psychiatric Nursing Care of the Adolescent Patient

Reading Assignment: Adolescent Psychiatric Nursing (Chapter 36)

Patient: Tiffany Sheldon, Pediatrics Floor, Room 305

Goal: To gain greater understanding of adolescence in order to provide psychiatric nursing care to an adolescent patient.

Objectives:

1. Understand the developmental stage of adolescence.
2. Explore select theoretical views of adolescence.
3. Identify key areas to include when assessing the adolescent patient.
4. Explore maladaptive responses seen in adolescence.
5. Describe effective nursing interventions when working with adolescents.
6. Explore the nurse's own issues when working with adolescent patients.
7. Evaluate expected treatment outcomes for an adolescent patient.

Exercise 1

Writing Activity

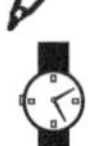

30 minutes

1. Adolescence is a unique stage of development when a shift in growth and learning occurs.

2. During adolescence, several important tasks must be accomplished before successfully transitioning into adulthood. List these tasks below.

mature relationships

accepting physical changes

marrage

3. Developmental tasks of adolescence are described in a variety of theories, from biological to moral. Using the biological theory, discuss the hormone and brain changes in adolescent development.

difference in hormone production

4. When conducting an assessment, the nurse must include key components specific to the adolescent patient, always checking for high-risk problems. Which of the following components are important to include for this special population? Select all that apply.

X Appearance

X Growth and development

X Parent and family health

X Emotional and physical status

X Coping and interaction patterns

X Activities of daily living

X Perception of health

X Family life

5. Adolescents think and worry about many issues. Which of the following issues is (are) typical of most adolescents?
   a. Body image
   b. Identity
   c. Independence
   d. Social role
   e. Sexual behavior
   f. All of the above
   g. Options a, c, and d only

6. Body image, identity, and independence are three issues that can produce adaptive or maladaptive responses as the adolescent attempts to cope with the developmental tasks at hand. Match each of these issues with the characteristics manifested during adolescence.

Adolescent Issue

B Body image

C Identity

A Independence

Characteristics

a. Seen as being free of parental control; seeks out adult situations; can become frightened and overwhelmed in the process

b. Wide variety of growth and development among age group; uneven and sudden growth common; compares self to peers

c. Childhood dreams end; becomes negative and contrary; can feel isolated, lonely, and confused

7. Maladaptive responses in adolescence include a variety of behaviors. Discuss the maladaptive responses of depression and body image.

absscence from school

poor grades

angry

substance abuse
Eating disorder

Exercise 2

Virtual Hospital Activity

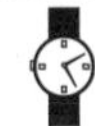

30 minutes

- Sign in to work at Pacific View Regional Hospital on the Pediatrics Floor for Period of Care 3. (*Note:* If you are already in the virtual hospital from a previous exercise, click on **Leave the Floor** and then on **Restart the Program** to get to the sign-in window.)
- From the Patient List, select Tiffany Sheldon (Room 305).
- Click on **Go to Nurses' Station**.
- Click on **Chart** and then on **305.**
- Click on and review the following chart sections: **History and Physical**, **Nursing Admission**, **Mental Health**, and **Consultations**.

1. In working with adolescents, the nurse must be able to distinguish between age-expected behavior and maladaptive responses. Based on your review of Tiffany Sheldon's chart, complete the table below and on the next page.

Issue in Adolescence	Age-Expected Behavior	Maladaptive Response
Body image	some issues because body is changing	lost weight instead of gaining weight
Mood	they think they are invinciable	Happy about weight loss

Issue in Adolescence	Age-Expected Behavior	Maladaptive Response
Activity	less physical activity	is in gynmastics

2. The specific problems that make Tiffany Sheldon a high-risk adolescent are:
   a. substance use and truancy.
   b. severe eating disorder and depressed mood.
   c. suicidal and self-injurious behavior.
   d. problems with conduct and violence.
   e. anxiety and sexual promiscuity.

3. The nurse must understand a few basic principles when working with adolescents. Identify the actions that represent the nurse's understanding of these principles in working with Tiffany Sheldon. Select all that apply.

   _X_ Meet individually with the patient to form an alliance and gain her perspective

   _X_ Provide health information about healthy and unhealthy adolescent activities

   _X_ Provide the adolescent with only written health information since she will be too embarrassed to listen to verbal information

   _X_ Educate the adolescent on normal teen behaviors

   ____ Only meet with the adolescent when the parents are also present

   _X_ Help the adolescent build healthy coping skills to deal with stress

4. Considering the psychological aspects of Tiffany Sheldon's maladaptive responses, discuss the types of therapy suggested in the Psychiatric Consult and the rationale for each therapy.

evaluation for depression
- help self esteem, body image, self-concept

Nutrition consult
- adequate fluid and electrolyte balances

5. Can you think of any of your own unresolved issues regarding adolescence that might arise if you were assigned to work with a patient such as Tiffany Sheldon? Explain.

friends on same diet?

how long she was on diet

Help see positives about self

6. The nurse must evaluate objectively the nursing care that has been provided to Tiffany Sheldon and her family. List the important questions to ask in determining whether Tiffany and her family have met the treatment goals outlined in the treatment plan.

food diary?

6 small calorie dense meals?

open with family?

Keep appropriate weight for height and age?

eating contract?

LESSON 14

Geropsychiatric Nursing Care

Reading Assignment: Geropsychiatric Nursing (Chapter 37)

Patient: Kathryn Doyle, Skilled Nursing Floor, Room 503

Goal: To understand, assess, and care for geriatric patients.

Objectives:

1. Identify symptoms of mental illness in older adults.
2. Discuss theories of aging from a variety of perspectives.
3. List specialized skills of the geropsychiatric nurse.
4. Acknowledge biases in working with older adult patients.
5. Provide a comprehensive assessment of the geriatric patient.
6. Describe common responses older adults have in relation to the aging process.
7. Plan and coordinate the care for a geriatric patient.
8. Identify effective treatment strategies to use with the geriatric patient and the patient's family.
9. Evaluate the care given to the geriatric patient.

Exercise 1

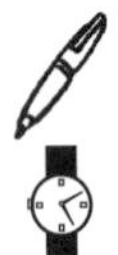

Writing Activity

15 minutes

1. Mental illness in older adults may be underestimated and left undiagnosed because the symptoms may be attributed to physical disorder, normalaging, cognative impairment, or the lack of age appropriate diagnostic criteria. For example, mental illnesses such as depression and anxiety are often misdiagnosed or undertreated.

2. Mental health in late life depends on a number of factors. Select all the factors that apply.

   X Physiological and psychological status

   X Economic resources

   X Social support systems

   X Personality

   X Typical lifestyle

3. The biological, psychological, and sociocultural theories of aging provide ways of defining aging and help to explain the causes and consequences of the aging process. Complete the table below and on the next page by summarizing these three theories.

Theory of Aging	Summary of Theory
Biological	gentic, symptomatic, cellular approach consequence of aging wear and tear on cells

Theory of Aging	Summary of Theory
Psychological	life development personality change can indicate brain disease
Sociocultural	individual & the environment age can change tolerance on the environment

4. Describe the specialized skills of the geropsychiatric nurse.

They need the skills oh psychiatric nursing & geriatric nursing

5. Case management is an especially effective approach to providing for the advacocy + protection needs of older adults.

6. Discuss any biases you may have in working with the geriatric population.

They are old, push overs, they smell

Exercise 2

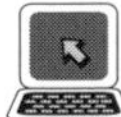

Virtual Hospital Activity

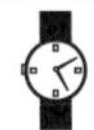

60 minutes

- Sign in to work at Pacific View Regional Hospital on the Skilled Nursing Floor for Period of Care 2. (*Note:* If you are already in the virtual hospital from a previous exercise, click on **Leave the Floor** and then on **Restart the Program** to get to the sign-in window.)
- From the Patient List, select Kathryn Doyle (Room 503).
- Click on **Go to Nurses' Station**.
- Click on **Chart** and then on **503**.
- Click on and read the **History and Physical**.
- Click on **Consultations** and read the Psychiatric Clinical Nurse Specialist Consult.

1. Kathryn Doyle has one of the four Ds of geropsychiatric assessment. Identify which one she has and discuss the need to include this issue in a geropsychiatric assessment.

depression, treat her with meds

2. Kathryn Doyle seems to be experiencing anxiety. Which of the following statements are true regarding anxiety in older adults? Select all that apply.

_____ Comorbid anxiety and depression are common in older adults.

_____ All types of anxiety combined are more prevalent than depression in older adults.

__X__ Untreated anxiety can contribute to sleep problems, cognitive impairments, and decreased quality of life.

_____ Anxiety does not affect the family.

__X__ Antianxiety medications also decrease depression.

3. Besides interviewing the geriatric patient and completing a mental status, there are other key components of the geropsychiatric nursing assessment. Complete the table below to include data specific to Kathryn Doyle.

Component	Key Elements	Assessment of Kathryn Doyle
Behavioral responses	depression	inmobility + loss of independence
Functional abilities	full ability: eating, writing, telephone, taking meds Some assistance: dressing, ambulation, toileting, bathing, laundry full assistnce: cooking cleaning, Shopping	
Physiological responses	needs a walker, hip fracture, depression	
Social support	small support	

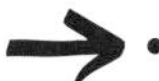

- Click on **Return to 503**.
- Click on **Patient Care** and then on **Nurse-Client Interactions**.
- Select and view the video titled **1150: Assessment—Depression**. (*Note:* Check the virtual clock to see whether enough time has elapsed. You can use the fast-forward feature to advance the time by 2-minute intervals if the video is not yet available. Then click again on **Patient Care** and **Nurse-Client Interactions** to refresh the screen.)

4. Depression and sadness are sometimes viewed as a normal part of aging. Kathryn Doyle's response to life events that have occurred over the past 9 months has resulted in a disturbance in her mood. In the list below, identify each true statement pertaining to normal sadness, grief, and loss in older adults. Select all that apply.

_____ Depression, grief, and loss are common in later life.

__X__ Prolonged grief and mourning need to be treated.

_____ Death of a life partner can compound the cumulative losses of aging.

__X__ The loss of hope by older adults with disabilities may result from or cause a depressive reaction.

__X__ Common symptoms of depression include decreased appetite and weight loss.

__X__ Fatigue, apathy, and loss of interest in friends and usual activities are symptoms of depression.

- Click on **MAR**.
- Review Kathryn Doyle's medication list.

5. Does Kathryn Doyle have medication ordered to treat her depression? Discuss the role of medication to treat depression in older adults.

No! decreases anxiety, promotes self-worth

6. Based on the nurse's assessment, Kathryn Doyle has other affective, somatic, stress, and behavioral responses common to older adults. Complete the table below by outlining her specific issues associated with these common reactions.

Type of Response	Specific Response	Issues Involved with Kathryn Doyle's Response
Affective	Situational low self-esteem	loss of independance
Somatic	Imbalanced nutrition	She can't go to the store and can't cook for herself
Stress	Relocation stress syndrome	has to live with son, girlfriend, + their son
Behavioral	Social isolation	unable to leave home

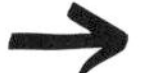

- Click on **Return to Nurses' Station**.
- Click on **Leave the Floor**.
- Click on **Restart the Program**.
- Sign in to work at Pacific View Regional Hospital on the Skilled Nursing Floor for Period of Care 3. Select Kathryn Doyle as your patient.
- Click on **Go to Nurses' Station**.
- Click on **503** at the bottom of the screen.
- Click on **Patient Care** and then on **Nurse-Client Interactions**.
- Select and view the video titled **1505: Assessment—Elder Abuse**. (*Note:* Check the virtual clock to see whether enough time has elapsed. You can use the fast-forward feature to advance the time by 2-minute intervals if the video is not yet available. Then click again on **Patient Care** and **Nurse-Client Interactions** to refresh the screen.)

7. Elder neglect and abuse has become more common in our society as older adults no longer have the status of respect they once had. Serving as the patient's advocate, the nurse must be on alert for signs of elder neglect, abuse, or exploitation. What are the signs that Kathryn Doyle is being neglected, exploited, or abused?

   avoidance, afraid son will be mad

8. During the family conference, the issue of theft will be addressed. Another concern that needs to be discussed is Kathryn Doyle continuing to live in her son's home after discharge. If this living arrangement is to work, the environment must include several basic characteristics that are therapeutic for older adult patients. In the list below, identify the critical elements that must be included in the environment. Select all that apply.

   _X_ Sense of calm and quiet

   _X_ Structured routine (based on the older adult's usual lifestyle)

   _X_ Consistent physical layout

   _X_ Activities that produce cognitive stimulation

   _X_ Safe environment

   _X_ Personal items that provide familiarity and a sense of security

   _X_ Focus on strengths and abilities

9. Most older adults (about 85%) are cared for in the home. What topics should the nurse include in family education and support sessions that would be critical to Kathryn Doyle's recovery and future?

- patient security
- resources for meds
- aging process

10. Aftercare for older adult patients is often necessary for a successful treatment outcome. After discharge, what agency support do you think Kathryn Doyle's son will need in the care of his mother in the home?

home care nurse

living aid

assisted living facility

LESSON 15

Nursing Care of Survivors of Abuse and Violence

Reading Assignment: Care of Survivors of Abuse and Violence (Chapter 38)

Patient: Dorothy Grant, Obstetrics Floor, Room 201

Goal: To care for a patient who is a survivor of abuse and violence.

Objectives:

1. Identify characteristics of someone who has experienced abuse or violence.
2. Define characteristics common to violent families.
3. Discern between myths and realities associated with survivors of abuse.
4. Compare and contrast the Paternalistic Model and the Empowerment Model of intervention in relation to battered women.
5. Identify strengths and coping strategies of someone who is experiencing abuse or violence.
6. Discuss nursing assessment and interventions using the Empowerment Model.
7. Identify central themes in abusive relationships.
8. Understand common barriers to battered spouses leaving the abusive relationship.
9. Describe critical elements of a discharge plan of someone who is being abused.

Exercise 1

Writing Activity

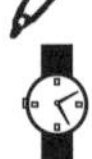

15 minutes

1. In describing someone who has experienced abuse or violence, provide a rationale for using the term *survivor* rather than *victim*.

2. Factors common to violent families include which of the following? Select all that apply.

    _____ Multigenerational family process

    _____ Owning and keeping weapons in the home

    _____ Social isolation

    _____ Use and abuse of power

    _____ Alcohol and drug abuse

3. Many myths exist regarding survivors of abuse. Complete the table below and on the next page by describing the reality associated with each myth listed.

Myth	Reality
Abused spouses can end the violence by divorcing their abuser.	

Myth	Reality
The abused partner can learn to stop doing things that provoke the violence.	
Being pregnant protects a woman from being battered.	
Abused women tacitly accept the abuse by trying to conceal it, not reporting it, or failing to seek help.	

4. The attitudes that nurses bring to the health care setting shape their responses toward survivors of violence. Which of the following statements are true? Select all that apply.

_____ Nurses may blame the survivor if behavior leading up to the abuse was questionable.

_____ Nurses often have difficulty understanding why a battered woman does not leave her abuser.

_____ Nurses always believe that people get what they deserve.

_____ Nurses may offer advice and sympathy instead of respect.

_____ The more the patient resembles the nurse, the easier it is for the nurse to recognize violence.

_____ More nurses have been victimized by violence than have any other work group.

_____ Nurses need to forget about their own experiences with violence.

_____ Nurses who have had clinical experiences with survivors of violence may be less likely to blame than nurses who have not.

5. What is your attitude about domestic violence, and how is it shaped?

Exercise 2

Virtual Hospital Activity

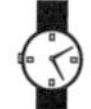

30 minutes

- Sign in to work at Pacific View Regional Hospital on the Obstetrics Floor for Period of Care 2. (*Note:* If you are already in the virtual hospital from a previous exercise, click on **Leave the Floor** and then on **Restart the Program** to get to the sign-in window.)
- From the Patient List, select Dorothy Grant (Room 201).
- Click on **Go to Nurses' Station**.
- Click on **Chart** and then on **201**.
- To answer questions 1 through 6, review the following sections of Dorothy Grant's chart: **Nursing Admission**, **Mental Health**, and **Consultations**. (*Hint:* In the Mental Health section, read the Psychiatric/Mental Health Assessment; then scroll down to review the Abuse Screening.)

1. Listed below are the five forms of abuse within families that reflect domestic struggles for power and control. Which form(s) is Dorothy Grant experiencing? Select all that apply.

   _____ Physical

   _____ Sexual

   _____ Emotional

   _____ Psychological

   _____ Economic

2. Dorothy Grant is a member of one of the special populations that are vulnerable to abuse. These populations include children, older adults, and developmentally disabled individuals, as well as ____. The most widespread form of family violence is abuse of ____.

3. General characteristics of violent families are listed in the left column below. In the right column, identify any specific characteristics of Dorothy Grant's family that correspond to the general characteristics of violent families.

Characteristic of Violent Families	Dorothy Grant's Family Characteristics
Multigenerational transmission	
Social isolation	
Use and abuse of power	
Alcohol and drug abuse	

4. What are Dorothy Grant's strengths in dealing with her abusive situation?

5. What are Dorothy Grant's coping strategies in dealing with her abusive relationship?

6. Depression is a common response by women in abusive relationships. According to Dorothy Grant's depression scale, her level of depression is ______________________.

Exercise 3

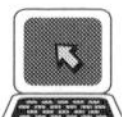

Virtual Hospital Activity

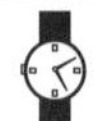

30 minutes

- Sign in to work at Pacific View Regional Hospital on the Obstetrics Floor for Period of Care 2. (*Note:* If you are already in the virtual hospital from a previous exercise, click on **Leave the Floor** and then on **Restart the Program** to get to the sign-in window.)
- From the Patient List, select Dorothy Grant (Room 201).
- Click on **Go to Nurses' Station**.
- Click on **201** at the bottom of the screen.
- Click on **Patient Care** and then on **Nurse-Client Interactions**.
- Select and view the video titled **1115: Nurse-Patient Communication**. (*Note:* Check the virtual clock to see whether enough time has elapsed. You can use the fast-forward feature to advance the time by 2-minute intervals if the video is not yet available. Then click again on **Patient Care** and **Nurse-Client Interactions** to refresh the screen.)

1. The Empowerment Model of intervention has been found to be very effective in working with battered women. The basic principles of this model are listed below and on the next page. In the video you just viewed, the nurse used the Empowerment Model when interacting with Dorothy Grant. In the right column below and on the next page, cite specific examples of statements made by the nurse that correspond to the Empowerment Model's principles. (*Note:* You may add suggestions of what the nurse *could have said* to support the Empowerment Model if you think there is room for improvement.)

Empowerment Model	Nurse's Statements
There is a mutual sharing of knowledge and information.	
The nurse strategizes with the survivor.	

Empowerment Model	Nurse's Statements
Survivors are helped to recognize societal influences.	
The survivor's competence and experience are respected.	

2. The nurse uses other therapeutic responses when interacting with Dorothy Grant. These are listed in the right column below. Match each response to the technique being used by the nurse.

	Technique	Nurse's Response
_____	Mutual goal sharing	a. Offers active listening responses such as "Feeling scared is a perfectly normal reaction."
_____	Focusing	b. "The clinical nurse specialist and the social worker work together to identify your immediate needs."
_____	Using broad open-ended questions	c. "Right now, your first priority is your own well-being and the well-being of your children."
_____	Listening	d. "Would you like to talk about your concerns now?" and "Is there anything I can do to help?"

3. The immediate goal of the nurse in working with Dorothy Grant is to develop trust. To do this, the nurse must express nonjudgmental listening and psychological support. How did the nurse accomplish this (or not accomplish this) in the video?

4. Which of the following constraints will make it difficult for Dorothy Grant to leave her husband? Select all that apply.

_____ She is still in love with her husband.

_____ She has a lack of housing and financial resources.

_____ Her church has a strong support of marriage.

_____ There is societal stigma against a woman who leaves her husband.

_____ Domestic violence reporting is not mandatory in any state.

_____ Her husband is in jail.

5. Dorothy Grant has left her husband twice before and returned. For the battered woman, what are the three main purposes of this behavior?

6. One of the most frightening realities Dorothy Grant may face in leaving her husband is

____.

7. Several themes expressed by women in abusive relationships have been identified. Knowing the themes Dorothy Grant is expressing will help the nurse in assessing and planning interventions. Identify Dorothy Grant's specific themes below.

Themes of Women Who Have Been in Abusive Relationships	Dorothy Grant's Themes
Lack of relational authenticity	
Immobility	
Emptiness	
Disconnection	

8. Discharge planning will be crucial for Dorothy Grant. Which of the following activities will be necessary for a successful outcome? Select all that apply.

_____ Create a safety planning checklist.

_____ Provide her with survivors of abuse and violence hotline phone numbers.

_____ Find a supportive alternate living arrangement for Dorothy Grant and her children.

9. Discuss your own thoughts about Dorothy Grant's current and past responses to the abuse. Do you think she has responded in the way a typical person would react to incredible physical and emotional trauma? Or do you believe her responses have been more pathological in nature? Explain.